SLEEP THIEF, restless legs syndrome

A guide to the current treatment and ways to cope for those whose sleep and ability to sit quietly are mysteriously stolen every evening. Although written for the lay public and victims of RLS, it may also be of interest to physicians who are baffled by this rest robber.

Virginia N. Wilson

Arthur S. Walters, M.D., Editor

SLEEP THIEF, restless legs syndrome

Virginia N. Wilson

with
David Buchholz, M.D.
Giorgio Coccagna, M.D.
Bruce Ehrenberg, M.D.
Mark Flapan, Ph.D.
Wayne A. Hening, M.D., Ph.D.
Alan Kanter, M.D.
Elio Lugaresi, M.D.
Jacques Montplaisir, M.D., Ph.D., FRCP
Ralph Pascualy, M.D.
Daniel Picchietti, M.D.
J. Steven Poceta, M.D.
Frankie Roman, M.D.
Lawrence Scrima, Ph.D.
Claudia Trenkwalder, M.D.
Arthur S. Walters, M.D.

edited by Arthur S. Walters, M.D.

—

Galaxy Books, Inc.
Orange Park, Florida

Galaxy Books, Inc.
Post Office Box 1421
Orange Park, FL 32067

First Edition
Publisher: Galaxy Books, Inc.
Cover Design: Jefferson Rall, Robin Shepherd Studio
Production: Paul Delage
Editorial Assistance: Kathleen Delage

Jane Brody Quote ©Copyright 1996 The New York Times Co. Published by permission.

Library of Congress Catalog Card Number: 96-76822
ISBN 0-9652682-0-9 Soft Cover
ISBN 0-9652682-1-7 Hard Cover

DEDICATION

I dedicate this book to the memory of Oron F. Hawley (1899 - 1996). It has been said that one person can change the world. Certainly Oron changed the world for all of us who suffer from restless legs syndrome (RLS). Oron and I never met face to face, but in spite of the thousands of miles between us, we were friends who had one common bond, a mysterious malady. In January 1990 he wrote the simple important-to-me line, "You are not alone, Virginia." Together we learned many other people also suffer. Although Oron did not participate in the forming of the RLS Foundation, he gave moral and financial support to it until the time of his death, just a few weeks short of his 97th birthday. His wanting to help others inspired me to spread the word that RLS is a physical and treatable disorder.

This dedication would not be complete without naming Pickett Guthrie, who also suffers with restless legs, as a living example of one person who can change the world. She has changed the lives of countless RLS victims. The RLS Foundation has flourished under her wisdom and personable business acumen. With her leadership, RLS has found its rightful place in the medical world. This book is a "thank you" for her selfless devotion.

Virginia N. Wilson
Orange Park, Florida 1996

Author's note

Restless Legs Syndrome (RLS) can be a serious disorder. Some 12 million Americans (and millions more throughout the world) are afflicted to varying degrees of severity with this treatable, physical disorder. Persons suspecting that they may be afflicted with RLS or Periodic Limb Movements in Sleep (PLMS) should consult a qualified physician as soon as possible. This book concerning RLS and PLMS is offered for informational purposes only, and should not be considered a substitute for the advice of a qualified physician.

The opinions expressed by those contributing to the text have been given freely. Each author has chosen to write about one area of the study of RLS so that some information may be repeated now and then to stress a particular point of view. Mostly the specific names of medications have been eliminated except for the particular chapters devoted to the subject of medication. These have been carefully edited by Drs. Wayne Hening and Arthur S. Walters to ensure the information is correct. All medications mentioned must be prescribed by a physician.

The author, Virginia N. Wilson, has received written permission from each patient whose letters have been quoted. There has been no payment given for any quotation, nor for the chapters written by the doctors and the author.

Authors' Royalties from the sale of this book will go to the RLS Foundation to help others find their ways through the maze the restless legs syndrome creates.

Virginia N. Wilson
Orange Park, Florida 1996

Table of Contents

SECTION II

The Patient, the Doctor, and Medication

10 SLEEP THIEF, restless legs syndrome

Foreword and Introduction

Your Time Machine

So they catch you napping
and laugh when you nod
as you try to converse.
Those snatches of drifting sleep
replenish your nerves,
rekindle the fire in your engine,
steam-generate the sagging body,
steam-clean the sluggish brain
refusing to neutralize
sparkling red and green lights
and sonic whistles of the nights.

Do not wear a hair shirt
nor beat your breast in shame
for dastardly deeds you did –
or did not do;
nor inflame guilt
to haunt your sleeplessness.
The truth is –
somewhere along your lifeway
you blew a paper-thin gasket
on your time machine –
your computer scrambles the program
eight hours out of every twenty-four.
Virginia N. Wilson

FOREWORD

This book has been written as a guide for the lay person to understand the Restless Legs Syndrome (RLS). The diagnosis and treatment of RLS and its allied condition, Periodic Limb Movements in Sleep (PLMS), are covered as well as the latest developments in RLS and PLMS research. Throughout this book, chapters by notable physicians and clinical investigators from around the world are interspersed with chapters by patients. Most of these are written by the principal author, Virginia N. Wilson. It has been a pleasure to work with Virginia N. Wilson, a published poetess now in her early eighties, who has turned her vivid descriptive writings to the problem of RLS from which she also suffers. Throughout the many chapters she has written for the book are helpful suggestions and the kinds of personal observations that can only be gained from experience. She has received many letters from people with RLS and she has spent many a long night talking with them over the telephone in an attempt to give them some help and comfort. She gives us some sensitive portraits of these very real human beings undergoing very real human suffering.

In this book you will learn about the primary form of RLS. In addition, Dr. Steve Poceta from Scripps Clinic in La Jolla, California, has a chapter on the secondary forms of RLS such as those associated with peripheral nerve damage. Dr. Larry Scrima of The Sleep Alertness Disorder Center, Inc., Aurora, Colorado, and Dr. Ralph Pascualy of the Sleep Disorders Center, Providence Medical Center, Seattle, Washington, tell us of other sleep disorders that may be associated with RLS and PLMS. A cogent explanation of the relationship between RLS and PLMS is given by Dr. David Buchholz from the Johns Hopkins sleep group of Drs. Buchholz, Richard Allen, and Chris Earley. A description of mainstream medical therapy is given by Dr. Wayne Hening from our own group which is headed at Robert Wood Johnson Medical School and the Lyons VA Medical Center by Dr. Sudhansu Chokroverty. Dr. Alan Kanter of Irvine, California, describes alternative modes of therapy including vein sclerotherapy. Dr. Bruce Ehrenberg of Tufts, Boston and Dr. Claudia Trenkwalder of the Max-Planck Institute Munich, Germany, each share a chapter with me, one on the genetics of RLS and the other on the 24-hour variability of symptoms in RLS. RLS in children is described by Dr. Dan Picchietti of the Carle Clinic, Urbana, Illinois.

Dr. Frankie Roman, Director of the Center for Sleep Disorders, Massillon, Ohio, is both the physician who treats RLS and an RLS patient himself. His chapter "Being Both the Doctor and the Patient" provides helpful hints for RLS patients in any walk of life. Patient Carol Walker tells us how to break the "patient mode" and gain personal power over RLS by self education. Patient Thelma Bradt tells us about the organization of patient support groups such as those sponsored by the RLS Foundation. Patient Jeanne Schell tells us of the history of RLS. Bob Guthrie whose wife is an RLS sufferer and Executive Secretary of the RLS Foundation gives the "How to" of installing an exercise bike in a van. RLS is very common and Dr. Mark Flapan's article on "Living with a Rare Disorder" was not originally directed toward RLS patients. However, we are reprinting it here with permission since it provides much useful information on coping with a chronic disorder. Bob Balkam helped me complete the list of publications relating to RLS (Appendix 3).

Dr. Jacques Montplaisir of Montreal, is one of the world's most respected and experienced sleep clinicians and researchers. His exposure to RLS is extensive and he provides some interesting and unique insights into RLS in his chapter "Restless Legs Syndrome: The Canadian Experience."

Dr. Elio Lugaresi discovered the periodic nature of the "Periodic Limb Movements in Sleep" some thirty years ago. Still active as chairman of the Department of Neurology at the University of Bologna, Italy, he and his long time colleague Dr. Georgio Coccagna give us a close personal historical look at the thought processes and excitement of one of their many important discoveries.

Arthur S. Walters, M.D., Editor
New Brunswick, New Jersey 1996

INTRODUCTION

Why Did I Write *SLEEP THIEF, restless legs syndrome?*

by Virginia N. Wilson

Who is this thief who silently slips into the lives of victims to steal their sleep and eventually their ability to live normal lives; to sit quietly while reading or watching TV; to attend church, movies, or meetings; to ride in a car or airplane; to stay seated while dining in a restaurant; to remain in bed all night with a spouse and never feel that over-powering need to move – stand – walk – or explode?

Who is this thief, the fiendish source of sleep deprivation, who masquerades as the off-spring of insomnia to conceal its true identity? The restless legs syndrome, known as RLS, is the clever actor with a skittish name who begins his work on most victims as daylight darkens into night.

Who would believe that the internal demand to move could completely destroy a person, leaving only dark-circled, puffy eyes and weary bone-tired bodies as evidence? There are no scars, no braces, no bandages to identify this victim's pain. Family members cannot understand why the RLS victim dreads vacation time and seems to lack the energy to enjoy family pleasures like riding across town to the beach or a state park for a picnic. There is little empathy with the person who has to watch a movie from the back of the theater or listen to the last song and benediction in the narthex of the church while standing, stepping in place, left foot – right foot – left – right – wishing the minutes would speed as seconds instead of dragging hours.

Few sufferers seek professional help to stop the pacing in dim-lit rooms night after night while the household rests. The thief cleverly covers all demoniac tracks by instilling guilt into the victim. These are a few of the malevolent thoughts planted by that scheming sleep thief. Over the years I've repeated them to myself hundreds of times.

I'm too tired to sleep. My job wears me thin every day.
I drank too much coffee.
The house is too hot – or too cold .
I must have a terrible secret buried within me that will not let me rest.

Being alone and not knowing what to do, where to get help, or even having someone to believe that you have a real life-threatening problem are the great hurdles RLS sufferers must jump every day – demon-hurdles controlled by the *SLEEP THIEF*

As secretary of the RLS Foundation I share desperate phone calls and letters with women and men of all ages, races, and socioeconomic groups, from every corner of the United States, Massachusetts to California and Texas to Montana, and now from sufferers living in Canada, Australia, South America, and Europe. For these people I have written this book.

To inform the general public and the medical world that RLS is a treatable physical disorder, not common insomnia nor a figment of the imagination as many friends, family members, and doctors think it might be, this book may be a guide. The crazy, creepy feelings of the legs that will not let a victim rest, the involuntary demanding of movement that overpowers any mind-over-matter thinking, needs to be out in the open. Only RLS sufferers can understand that a twenty minute cross-town ride can become a nightmare.

When I learned that an estimated 12 million Americans suffer from this disorder to varying degrees of severity, I knew someone must tell the whole world that RLS victims are not hypochondriacs imagining ills. They are not psychotic. They are victims of a physical, treatable disorder with a mystery source and as yet no cure. The need for educating the general public and the medical world are the seeds of the need to write this book. It is my hope and dream that these pages will aid RLS victims in coping with their everyday lives until a cure to slay this demon is found.

RLS does not kill people as does cancer and heart diseases, but in serious cases, it kills the physical, social, and familial lives of all who are unlucky enough to be so plagued.

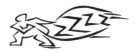

How I Became Interested in the Restless Legs Syndrome

by Arthur S. Walters, M.D., Editor
Chairman, RLS Foundation Medical Advisory Board

I first became interested in the restless legs syndrome (RLS) between 1982 and 1984 when Dr. Wayne Hening and I were Movement Disorder fellows together at the Neurological Institute – Columbia Presbyterian Medical Center in New York City. In 1983 we saw two patients with strange leg discomfort that made them walk the floor sleeplessly at night. They also had myoclonic twitching movements of the legs, awake and asleep. Both reported that their symptoms had serendipitously improved with opioids. Dr. Hening and I stayed up for two days and nights in a row studying the first patient, a difficult task since we had movement disorder rounds and clinics on both days. It was only later that we discovered Ekbom's description of Restless Legs Syndrome (RLS) and his casual mention of the possible opioid responsiveness of RLS. This began a more formal study of opioid treatment of RLS on our part and the rest, as they say, is history.

Dr. Hening and I subsequently obtained academic posts at the Department of Neurology, UMDNJ-Robert Wood Johnson Medical Center and its affiliate hospital, the Lyons VA Medical Center, where Dr. Sudhansu Chokroverty was, and still is, chief of Neurology. First as fellows and later as academics, we have explored new treatments for RLS such as the opioids, dopamine agonists like bromocriptine, and with Dr. Mary Wagner, adrenergic agents like clonidine. We have attempted to better define the clinical features of RLS. We have also explored the clinical features of a related form of motor restlessness, Neuroleptic-Induced Akathisia (NIA) and we have queried whether NIA may give clues to the cause of RLS. In addition, we have extended some of our therapeutic observations from RLS to NIA.

Many people have provided support and guidance along the way including Dr. Stan Fahn and Dr. Lucien Côtè of the Neurological Institute in New York, Dr. Neil Kavey of the Columbia Presbyterian Sleep Disorders Center in New York, and Dr. Sudhansu Chokroverty of UMDNJ-Robert Wood Johnson Medical School and Lyons VA Medical Center.

In addition to continuing to explore therapeutic options for RLS, we are currently involved in an attempt to find the gene for hereditofamilial RLS. We have collected blood samples from over 120 members in seven large families with RLS. The discovery of the gene and subsequently its biochemical product will essentially be the discovery of the cause of an important type of RLS. This in turn could lead us to newer and better therapies for RLS. Many authors of chapters in this book have contributed blood samples from RLS families for genetic analysis.

We have also organized an International Study Group for RLS composed of 28 scientists and doctors who are currently doing research on RLS. The first joint venture of the study group was to write a multi-authored paper entitled "Toward a Better Definition of the Idiopathic Restless Legs Syndrome" that was published in the journal *Movement Disorders* in 1995. Recently Dr. Claudia Trenkwalder came from the Max-Planck Institute, Munich. Germany, to the laboratory of Drs. Hening, Chokroverty, and myself to do a study on the circadian rhythmicity of RLS. The results of this study suggest that RLS is not only worse at night because patients are lying down more at this time, but also because of an independent biological factor with a regular 24 hour variation. This has important implications for the formulation of diagnostic criteria for RLS.

Other work of Drs. Hening, Chokroverty, and myself includes a retrospective study of the age of onset of RLS. One conclusion we have drawn from the study is that RLS has been previously underappreciated in childhood. The National RLS support group, "The Night Walkers," aided us in collecting data for this project. Also, we recently published the first full case reports of RLS in children. Collaboration is ongoing with Dr. Dan Picchietti of the Carle Clinic, Champaign-Urbana, Illinois, on the study of Attention Deficit Hyperactivity Disorder (ADHD) in children with RLS and Periodic Limb Movement Disorder (PLMD).

Community service has also been a major focus for us. The formation of the Restless Legs Syndrome Foundation (RLSF) or "Night Walkers," with its lay advisory board and attendant sixteen-member medical advisory board has been an important instrument in the education of both the public, patients, and medical community at large about RLS, its treatment, and its impact.

The principal author, Virginia Wilson, has dedicated this book to Oron Hawley and Pickett Guthrie. This book would not be complete without my own personal dedication to the late Karl A. Ekbom, M.D., who did the first extensive description of RLS in the 1940's.

Arthur S. Walters, M.D.
New Brunswick, New Jersey 1996

Acknowledgments by the Author

In 1992 Pickett Guthrie and I talked about the need for a book to help inform both the general public and the medical world about restless legs syndrome. With her encouragement the idea took form. When Dr. Arthur S. Walters offered his guidance and eagle eyed criticism of every word written for the book I believed *SLEEP THIEF, restless legs syndrome* could be achievable.

I am indebted to Dr. Walters for having faith in my project and for reading every word and editing every page. We both thank all those who wrote portions of the book: Doctors David Buchholz, Giorgio Coccagna, Bruce Ehrenberg, Mark Flapan, Wayne A. Hening, Alan Kanter, Elio Lugaresi, Jacques Montplaisir, Ralph Pascualy, Daniel Picchietti, J. Steven Poceta, Frankie Roman, Lawrence Scrima, and Claudia Trenkwalder plus Robert L. Guthrie and members of the RLS Board of Directors Robert M. Balkam, Thelma E. Bradt, Jeanne M. Schell, and Carol U. Walker.

I have never forgotten Elmer E. Hartgerink's surprising me with funds to start the book and my friends Arthur and Lora Bolte who, early on, sent a check to help with secretarial expenses. I want to thank all the Night Walkers who have been such an inspiration for me from the beginning and who gave me permission to use portions of their letters as quotes throughout the book. Indeed in early 1990 the little band of RLS sufferers who shared meager information with Oron Hawley and me did not dream that we were at the threshold of such an important venture into the medical world.

Most of all I want to express my gratitude to Kathy and Paul Delage who have shown great support for this project from the beginning and who made the book become a reality with their skills and hard work.

Last but not least, how can I ever thank my husband Jack for all the hours of neglect he has endured while this project was being born and nurtured?

Virginia N. Wilson
Orange Park, Florida 1996

Section I

The Restless Legs Syndrome and Other Sleep Disorders

What is sleep?

O magic sleep! O comfortable bird,

That broodest o'er the troubled sea of the mind

Till it is hush'd and smooth!

"Endymion," John Keats [1818]

The greatest minds of every era have studied the mystery of sleep. Some ancient people believed the soul wandered while the body rested, some thought sleep was a half-way state between life and death or that sleep was a curse casting a magic spell to take away the body's strength. Others believed wisdom and strength came with the magic of sleep. The truth is, no one has ever unraveled the mystery of the what and the why of sleep.

No one has a positive answer as to the reason for sleep, but there are abundant negative proofs that lost sleep leaves a person devastated, unable to perform at top rate, and a danger to himself and others. Researchers agree that people require at least eight hours of sleep, one-third of our allotted twenty four.

What happens to the missing one-third of each day of the RLS victim?

Chapter One

Do I have Witch's Blood in my Veins?: My Experience with RLS
by Virginia N. Wilson

Sometimes, at night, when my legs demand to move and force me to rise from my bed to walk alone in the dark house, I wonder if my husband's joking words, about my having witch's blood in my veins, might be true. I am a victim of the restless legs syndrome (RLS).

If you have not been properly introduced to this Sleep Thief, who steals from victims the pleasure of living a normal life, it is time for me to present the rest robber to you. This sneaky character arouses annoying, tickling sensations in the legs, and sometimes in the arms, which forces a victim to move, whether he or she wants to move or not. The Sleep Thief offers no choice! Walk or explode! Walking, even standing while marching in place, does calm those jittery feelings — temporarily — but, when the victim sits or lies down again, the urgency to move returns, with a vengeance.

My husband's referring to witch's blood began years ago when we noticed my restlessness occurred at night. Of course! What other time would a Sleep Thief work except when the sun disappears and shadows darken the landscape? The thief steals into our homes, into our living rooms or our bedrooms, to tease and torture unwitting victims.

Too few people are aware of the viciousness of this thief masquerading under the frivolous name "restless legs syndrome." How many times have we heard, "If you'd lie still when you go to bed you'd go to sleep"? Lie still? That's the problem! We can't sit or lie still. We spend a lifetime going from doctor to doctor seeking help. Sometimes we are labeled as a hypochondriac by the doctor, our families, and friends.

You, your mate, or dear friend may be one of those who believe they suffer with chronic insomnia. But the truth is, one of you may be a victim of the Sleep Thief, the mischief maker who plagues an estimated 12 million Americans each night.

I ask you to come share this typical nightly drama played out in countless homes by someone, who perhaps, unknowingly, suffers from RLS. Join me as night shadows envelop the house. It is time for Betty and Al to come for an evening of cards. I sit down to watch TV while I wait and almost immediately the creepy, crawly sensations sweep over my legs. I am forced to get on my feet — and walk to relieve them.

Our guests arrive. "Well, how did you like the new doctor?" Betty asks as she walks in the door.

Without missing a step I sigh, "Would you believe that he laughed at me?"

Betty looks at me sharply, "Laughed — at you? You must be kidding."

"I'm serious. He just laughed when I told him I couldn't sleep, that I couldn't hold my legs still at night, that I felt like I would explode if I didn't get up and walk. He said I was just imagining that since I knew I wouldn't explode."

Betty joins me and together we walk around the living and dining rooms, into the hall and back again.

"Did you tell him you can't ride in a car very far without your legs making you want to jump out and run?" Betty asks. I nod and Betty goes on, "Surely he came up with some solution."

"Oh, he did. Said I was suffering from stress. Believe me, I was stressed to the limit. I had been spilling my pain out and I don't think he listened to a word. He looked over my list of medications that all the doctors have had me try with no luck. He hummed a little m-m-m . . and said, 'Looks like you've tried about everything. Definitely shows you have a history of depression.'

"'My problem is I can't sleep,' I said. 'I seem to have to walk all night long even though I am so tired I can hardly drag one foot after the other.' And he looked up and repeated parrot-like, 'You can't sleep! Hm-m-m-m.' I hate it when someone, especially a doctor, goes hm-m-m. I quickly lose confidence because I know that person doesn't know what to say."

Betty nods agreement.

"'So you've had this sleeping problem many years?' he asked as he looked up, 'Could be your body doesn't require much sleep.' I just looked at him in dismay. That man didn't understand the first thing that I had said.

"He poked around, you know how they do — I think it makes them feel important. Maybe it is an act to impress the patient. He attached his stethoscope to his ears and listened here and there. He poked in my ribs and across my back, and said, 'Perhaps there is something pressing — we need to have a brain scan.' His voice trailed off as he reached for a small printed pad.

"'I had one, three months ago and everything was normal,' I said. 'The report should be in the file my doctor sent.' He shuffled the papers in the thin folder, shrugged and mumbled something like 'Oh, here it is.' He glanced over it, then we went into the old routine of touch your nose with your left forefinger . . . now your right . . . the rubber mallet on the knees . . . on and on — you know the same old stuff I've been doing for doctors all these years. He put a pin in my foot. 'Did you feel that, Mrs. Wilson?' he asked. Did I feel that? Of course I did!

"Again I asked him, 'Why do my legs get jumpy whenever I sit or lie down? I can't control them no matter how much I try and the harder I try to keep them quiet the wilder they get.' He laughed. He laughed! Can you imagine that? I asked a simple question about why couldn't I control my legs like any normal person should and he laughed.

"This really made me angry because I had come to this 'expert' who was supposed to know why I couldn't sleep, the one to whom my own doctor had sent me for help. Oh boy, I knew I had another one who didn't know what was wrong with me and didn't want to admit that he didn't know. He was grabbing at a straw when he announced with a positive tone in his voice, 'You're suffering from stress.'

"'You bet I am,' I said, 'You'd be stressed too if you had to survive on one or two or no hours of sleep every night.' Then he said, 'Perhaps you are working too hard, probably worrying too much. You need a rest.' I nodded. He finally got the picture.

"'That's what I'm here for,' I agreed. 'I need to rest. All I want is a simple night's sleep all in one piece — maybe even six hours.'

"'You may have some deep secret imbedded in your mind. Something so stressful your mind does not want to deal with it. I think it worth your while to have some sessions with a therapist recommended by a psychiatrist. You may be able to clear the conflict with your subconscious and then be able to sleep.'

"He scribbled a name and address of a psychiatrist on a prescription pad and handed me the paper. I was furious by this time. This 'expert' was charging me an arm and a leg and he didn't even know what I was talking about. I was trying to tell him about the creepy, crawly legs that keep me awake but he didn't want to listen. Stress was the only excuse he could give.

"I gathered up my purse and sweater and started toward the door Over my shoulder I said, 'I've already been to a psychiatrist, a hypnotist, an acupuncturist, a chiropractor. You name it, I've tried it. I don't think you're going to help me either.'

"He walked to the door with me and said, 'Stress can be a physical, chemical, or emotional factor that causes bodily or mental tension and may be a factor in disease causation'

"'So does lack of sleep,' I answered and walked out."

"Good for you! I just can't imagine a doctor laughing at a patient," Betty says shaking her head slowly.

Jack calls out, "Enough of this doctor talk. Come on, let's play cards. Personally I think Virginia has witch's blood in her veins and needs to prowl all night." He sits down and begins dealing the cards. This is the signal that play is about to begin. No more woman chitchat allowed!

I spend over half the time Betty and Al are here, going in and out of the kitchen, pretending to check on the refreshments. I check the cheese cake in the refrigerator and busy myself rechecking the silver, plates and napkins already on the counter. Even those breaks aren't enough to relieve my restless legs. When I return to the living room I stand on one foot and then the other while playing, laughing a laugh I don't feel inside but I jabber on, "This way I can see your cards better. Maybe I'll win a game."

My inability to sit is well known by all my friends. They also know that my condition is worsening. I am experiencing more restlessness and difficulty in concentrating. It is obvious that I am having problems with keeping my mind on the cards being played.

I am relieved when the game is over and I joke, "With all those chances to cheat I still didn't win."

After Betty and Al leave, Jack turns to the eleven o'clock nightly news without comment. I try sitting on the sofa thinking I might lie back, listen, and rest. In less than a minute I have to pace again — around — around — between rooms, listening to the newscasters and the advertisements of cars and sports interspersed with music. I look out the window at the menacing blackness that enfolds the house. NIGHT! Sometimes I wish the sun would never set because with evening comes the agony between my skin and bones, up and down my legs.

Jack looks up as I make the turn across the room and laughs, "You know there's a full moon out tonight. Do you hear any werewolves? I've locked up the broom closet just in case you want to take off."

"That's what I feel like doing! Only I really feel like I'm going to explode!"

"Well, let me get out of the way." He laughs. Like an old time vaudeville act we've been doing this same routine for too many years. We both know that my lack of sleep and my need to walk are like thieves robbing me of rest and sleep — every night — stealing from us our normal lives. When the newscast ends, Jack turns off the reading lamp beside his chair and rises, and I stop pacing long enough to give him a quick hug and kiss. He walks down the long hall to his room . . . alone. Long ago my legs had jerked me out of our queen-size bed. I had kicked and turned so much he suggested separate rooms when we built our retirement home. It was fine with me, for the many years I couldn't count I had ended every night sleeping on the sofa in the living room. My lack of sleep had become a Damoclean sword hanging over our marriage.

Hopeful this night would be different, this night would grant me rest, I follow him down the pathway of small night-lights to my own room. We've lived with night lights in every corner of the house for years. Jack doesn't like them but the fear of falling over some shadowed misplaced article, while I walk the night hours away, has made me wary of a dark household.

We exchange "good nights" at our doorways and I go into my room. Jack doesn't understand how desperately tired I am all the time. He sleeps like a log every night. No thunderstorms bother him. Shrill fire-engine sirens can race by and not disturb his rest. Sometimes I am jealous of his gift of sleep, jealous and yet thankful that he is not plagued with my problem.

I slide into my single bed, pull the covers up to my neck, move the pillow, move it again. My eyes droop with weariness, but my legs do not receive a sleep message from my brain. I listen to Jack's regular, deep snore from across the hall. For so many years I have blamed him for keeping me awake, night after night and yet, in the darkness the snoring sound is comforting. Really soft, even, restful like water of a stream rushing over rocks. No, I can't blame Jack for my inability to sleep. There has to be another reason. Hadn't my day been full of activity — and yes, stress? My mind raced on. Maybe I really am crazy. Maybe I do have some deep dark secret hidden within me that will not let me rest. Maybe the doctor was right. Did some awful thing happen to me in my childhood that is so horrible it will not let me rest? Am I the only person in the world who can't sleep but must walk on and on?

I begin to pray, "Dear Lord . . . ." The words trail off into nothingness. My legs begin moving. Slowly each foot slides up and down, smoothing each leg, ankle to knee. Then they speed into side-to-side movement. I try to massage my calves and thighs into submission. Futile! Then comes the thrashing. Slowly I get up and walk down the dim-lit hall. I give up the fight and go looking for a pain pill, even though my legs don't pain. They don't ache. I hope for some kind of relief. If I could only find something to let me lie quietly! Rest! Even if I don't go to sleep.

"Maybe I'm hungry," I reason aloud. I know that is not true. Hadn't we had refreshments less than an hour ago?

"I don't need to eat anything," I whisper to myself as I enter the kitchen, look inside the refrigerator, rummage about until my fingers touch the pan with the remains of the cheese-cake topped with cherry sauce. The cake is delicious. I scrape the pie pan clean and lick the fork, and scold myself, whispering as though someone might hear.

"I shouldn't have done that. I'm adding pound after pound with this snacking every night. But somehow sweets make me feel better. Tomorrow I'll feel so guilty when Jack looks in the refrigerator then turns to me and says, 'So you ate the cheese cake last night after I went to bed! You know you shouldn't do that! I keep telling you that's why you can't sleep. You complain about having to walk all night.' He'll stomp out the door and call back, 'No need talking to you about it. You never learn!'"

I wash the dish and fork, wipe them, put them away to hide my guilt-ridden episode. I hope that Jack won't notice my raiding the refrigerator this time. It is so hard to explain to him this feeling of near hysteria. The endless searching for something to help — anything. I snap off the over-the-counter light and walk into the living room.

The bridge table with its four vacant chairs is at the far end of the room. I deal a hand of solitaire and hope I can sit long enough to play a game. "One-two-three-four-five-six-seven-eight-nine-ten. One-two-three — " It helps to count aloud. The sound of my voice is comforting in the vacant room. I can't sit. I stand and continue to deal. "One-two-three — ." I sit then stand a while, alternating as my legs demand. I miss plays, confuse clubs with spades and hearts with diamonds. An hour passes. I don't win the first game, nor the second. It doesn't matter. Slowly my legs feel a slight numbness, a hint of sleep. I leave the cards scattered over the table top and feel my way along the dim, familiar hall, hoping this time I can stay in bed for at least three or four hours. Five would be better.

As I pass a window I peer at the outer, unfriendly, impenetrable darkness. I wonder how many miles I've walked since sundown. A 26 mile marathon? I feel like it. Whatever is plaguing me holds tightly and does not want to let me go. What have I done to cause this? What is stealing my sleep every night and why? Like a slow, dreamy sleep walker, I crawl into bed. Tears seep from the corners of my eyes.

"Maybe I do have witch's blood in my veins like Jack says."

Exhaustion sweeps over me. I sleep for two hours. Dawn sends stabs of light through my eyelids. I moan, "Another day — and I just got to sleep!"

Chapter Two

Dancing on Fred Astaire Legs – *Not Willingly*:
The Joy of Finding Help.

by Virginia N. Wilson

I muddled through the 1985 Christmas holidays like a zombie. For weeks my sleep time had diminished. Even sitting in a tub of warm water didn't help. Night after night found me wandering into our empty living room, turning on the TV. Dimmed shadows crept over the monitor and splattered alternating white and gray mixed with splashes of brilliant color over the walls and furniture. Often my walking accelerated into dancing on Fred Astaire legs – not willingly – not gracefully. As the pressure increased, I began my version of the Mexican Hat Dance, stamping furiously left foot, right foot, left foot, around a make-believe broad brim of a straw hat like the many I'd seen when we had traveled in that land south of the border.

Uncontrollably, my feet stamped like I might be stepping on fire ants rushing to attack me. Furiously, I flew about the feigned hat brim and then, as if by magic, I began to feel my muscles relax. My legs quieted and slowly I moved down the hall toward my bedroom.

This went on night after night. No one, friends, family, or physician believed me when I said that I didn't sleep at all. But my daytime reactions proved to me that my body was completely sleep deprived. Often I fell asleep while trying to eat and my head fell face-down into my filled plate, waking me up immediately. I sat in armed chairs to keep me from falling sideways onto the floor. I took a walk one morning and I fell asleep and crashed to the sidewalk. Fortunately, I only skinned my nose and chin. My dignity suffered as neighbors rushed out to help me find my broken glasses.

While driving to the doctor's office I fell asleep at the wheel, drove up over the curbing. What if there had been a group of children on that corner when my car jumped that curb? I was frantic! At that moment I knew I had hit the bottom of my wellness well. There was no more strength, no more ability to live a normal life left in me. My doctor was compassionate but couldn't help. Together we had tried everything he could think of or read about.

That evening I phoned my son in New York City and told him of my disaster.

"Mom, you've got to get help. Come up here and go through the sleep lab at Cornell University." (There were few sleep clinics at that time and I had never thought about going to one.) "One of my friends worked there and said it was very pleasant and they do a good job. I'm sure they can find out why you can't sleep. There's got to be a reason!"

"It's a long way from Florida to New York. I don't think I can sit that long in a plane."

"Don't come non-stop. Make several stops along the way, then you can get out and walk," he argued.

He gave me the phone number to call for making an appointment at the sleep center in White Plains and wouldn't take no for an answer.

"Okay," I said, too tired to argue. That turned out to be the best "Okay" I ever said.

My doctor agreed that this was a good move, as he was worried about my condition. He sent my personal records ahead to be examined by the clinic staff. After two weeks of filling out sleep pattern papers for the clinic, I boarded a plane with no medication to take to ease my anxiety. The plane made several stops along the way and I did get out and walk.

My son and his wife met me at the airport. We had dinner, went to a stage play (which I watched from the back of the theater while I jumped up and down). Frankly, I don't even remember what we saw or where we ate. I was absolutely miserable trying very hard to act like a civilized human being. It's hard when you really want to scream and run or dance a jig in the street. We rode the train to White Plains and the cab driver told my son that the last train back to New York would be returning within a few minutes. I was literally dumped on the curbing of a just opened hotel. Building supplies seemed to be everywhere. I went to my room to walk or play solitaire all night. The hospital was only a few blocks away. I walked to my nine a.m. appointment. The air was cold and invigorating. I dismissed my tiredness. I find that RLS sufferers can do that very successfully. We seem to garner energy whenever it is needed. That is one of our difficulties. No one believes that we have a disabling disorder.

The hospital looked like a library, not a hospital as I think of one, all glass and marble. It was delightfully old with wood paneled walls and young people scurrying around. I spent most of the day with neurologists, answering questions to help the staff decide if I were a qualified candidate for a full sleep test. I was. I was dismissed until nine p.m. when my sleep adventure would begin.

I tried to shop in the exclusive shops surrounding the area but weariness swept over me and I barely made it back to the hotel room to collapse on the bed, but not to sleep. I ate in the hotel dining room, then walked back to the hospital with a small packet of sleep wear. The floor was completely empty when I got off the elevator. Lights were dimmed, no students milled about. One room filled with monitors and desks was brightly lighted. I went to the door and a young man greeted me. It was time for the test to begin.

I was prepared for bed, I thought: pajamas, a robe, slippers. I was fitted with a harness of wires and plugs. Small electrodes were placed on my head. Wires wandered down my legs and arms. The young man took a Polaroid picture of me wearing my full regalia. I was ushered into a very comfortable bedroom, resembling a hotel room, complete with TV, radio, and private bath.

"Just call me with this button any time you need to get out of bed," the young man said. How he was going to get me out of bed with all this hardware attached was a mystery. How I would use the bathroom posed a problem.

I couldn't see him, but I knew he was there watching the little pen scratches on the monitor panel before him. He had shown me all the equipment before I had prepared for the night's test. How long could I stay in that bed without calling for help? Probably ten minutes at the most and I pushed the panic button. I was unhooked from the harness with a quick pull of a plug. I was free to walk except I had a lot of weighty hardware hanging on me. I have no idea how many times this young man came to my rescue. I walked up and down the dim lit halls dozens of times and he didn't even act upset. I got hungry. He made some oatmeal. I wanted a cup of coffee but he said no to that.

At last the night ended. I had an appointment with a doctor for nine o'clock. Not so. It snowed so much the good doctor couldn't get into the hospital. A mini-bus came and took a few stragglers like me out of the compound, back to the snow filled streets. I had to wait in the hotel for a whole day and another night for the results of the test.

That next morning Dr. Daniel Wagner introduced himself and after reviewing the papers filled with lines and squiggles he said, "You have the restless legs syndrome."

"The what?" I asked.

"Your legs move so much it is impossible for your body to go to sleep. I've already spoken to your physician and he said he had read about the restless legs syndrome in a medical journal where it was described but had no suggested medical therapy. We're going to keep in touch until we get you medicated properly. It can be done but it often takes time and a lot of trial and errors. Restless legs syndrome is a common sleep disorder but so few people, even doctors, recognize it as a problem."

My son sent a limousine for the ride back to the NY airport so that I might catch my flight home and I enjoyed every minute of the snow packed landscape but mostly I enjoyed knowing that I had a physical problem that had a real name. Simple as it may sound, I had the restless legs syndrome. What a relief to learn that I was not crazy, that I was not a hypochondriac as some people thought. While I didn't wish this affliction on anyone, it was comforting to know that I was only one among a lot of other people who were experiencing this same problem. I didn't sleep on the way home, but there was hope for sleep in my future, medication was waiting for me at the pharmacy. This was the dawning of a new era. I was determined to find all the available information about this physical disorder that had almost ruined my life.

Chapter Three

The Mysterious Robber of Sleep: Restless Legs Syndrome

by Virginia N. Wilson
Ralph Pascualy, M.D., contributor

Restless Legs Syndrome (RLS) is the most familiar name of the sleep thief but the disorder is listed in the J. B. Lippincott Company *Dictionary of Medical Syndromes, (Second Edition)* under many names: Wittmaack-Ekbom Syndrome; Anxietas tibialis; asthenia crurum paresthetica; Ekbom's; leg jitter; **restless legs**.

Symptoms: Recurrent, unpleasant, peculiar creeping or crawling sensation in the legs, occasionally in the thighs or feet, felt deep inside the muscle or bones, which prevents the patient from keeping the involved extremities still. Bilateral and symmetric involvement or preponderant on one side; seldom affecting the arms and hands in 'tono minor.' Seldom true pain. Worse in the evening and at night or when the patient rests for some time. Sometimes lasting only a short period, sometimes hours. Sensation is relieved by movement, but reappears a short time after patient returns to bed. Important cause of severe insomnia.

Add to the sensations referred to in the dictionary pulling, prickling, tingling, itching, or more colorful descriptions from letters written by RLS victims:

Like a toothache in my legs.

. . . with Pepsi-cola in my veins.

My aunt had RLS too and she said, "It felt like rats were crawling on my legs at night."

I have jumpy legs . . . I rock and roll for hours sometimes.

. . . tickling pain . . . difficult to explain . . . it is inside my bones and causes me to beat on my thighs.

as if the inside wants to get outside but there is no visible muscle twitching, cramping or movement apparent.

Dr. Ralph Pascualy[1] explains how RLS affects individuals in different ways:

> Restless legs is a feeling which is very hard to describe, and the words that people use to talk about it are often confusing to the doctor. It may be a pain. It may be an ache. It may be a crawling feeling like you have worms in your legs. It may be like a tiny set of itches or pin pricks. And because the words are so different from person to person, the physician may think it's simply a cramp, or maybe it's arthritis, maybe it's just nervousness, maybe it's one type of problem related to diabetes which causes changes in the nerves, or maybe it's due to loss of blood flow in the legs if the person is older. [So often the sensation is explained away by the patients themselves or by the doctor.]

---

[1] Dr. Ralph Pascualy, a Member of the RLSF Medical Advisory Board, and Medical Director of the Providence Sleep Disorders Center, in Seattle, Washington, gave an overview of related sleep problems on January 15, 1994, in a welcoming speech before the meeting of the Seattle Sleep Disorders Support Groups for patients with sleep apnea, narcolepsy, and restless legs syndrome.

But there is one interesting thing about restless legs which is only true of that problem: if you move or walk, the symptom gets much, much better or may go away. If you have arthritis, it does not go away by walking. It might even hurt you more. Or if you have a problem with diabetes that has damaged the nerves in your feet, that [usually] does not go away. In fact it is present all day. This discomfort, the medical word which is fancy and unhelpful, is dysesthesia which means you have a feeling you can't describe properly. If you have that and it goes away by moving your legs, you probably have restless legs.

Some victims experience a slow annoyance like a feather duster lightly skimming over the legs which may last for a short time or turn into a demand to stand and later to walk or dance about. The demand to move the legs, which sometimes become excessive, makes rational thinking difficult because nothing seems to be able to stop the senseless movements. While RLS is not life threatening, it can become dangerous when the body is completely out of control and the suffering seems unbearable. The urge to jump out of a moving car becomes obsessive. Even jumping from a sky-scraper window might seem to be one way out of a "what-can-I-do-to-stop-this?" moment.

We can laugh about doing the Mexican Hat dance but when a full attack comes over a victim such vigorous activity can become a reality – like trampling a sand mound to subdue fire ants. Perhaps the most troublesome is the speed with which the urge to move can and sometimes does become uncontrollable; but, the great joy is, it may stop just as rapidly as it began. There seems to be no reason for the beginning or the end of the action.

While this violent exercise is taking place the victim blames himself or herself for eating the wrong food for dinner, for wearing the wrong shoes, or for working too hard in the garden or at the office. The dancer believes sleep deprivation is the robber, and exhaustion causes a breakdown of the nervous system. The sleep robber contorts minds to believe his devilishness is an effect rather than the cause.   Victims conjure up excuses for this smooth scam-artist. "Jumpy, nervous, jittery legs" seldom are considered the cause of being unable to go to sleep or stay asleep if awakened.

While the origin of RLS is obscure, the disorder itself is very alive at the present time. It is estimated that up to 5% of our population (over 12 million Americans, and millions more throughout the world) may be suffering from it in various degrees of intensity, from occasional annoyances to daily severe attacks. Most cases of RLS are diagnosed for patients aged sixty or more years, yet we are finding more and more younger persons suffer severely during "prime earning years" and they have the added worries of job security along with the aggravations of unwanted movement and loss of sleep. Like many neurological disorders, psychological stress can aggravate RLS symptoms.

One of the greatest aggravations suffered by RLS victims is the lack of proper diagnosis. The purpose of this book is to make the public aware that this disorder is physical and treatable. We have too many physicians who do not acknowledge the existence of RLS. Nor do they recognize symptoms which require no expensive sleep disorder testing. Arthur S. Walters, M.D., Department of Neurology at the Robert Wood Johnson Medical School, gives this test to ascertain the presence of the restless legs syndrome.   Does the patient:

• Have "crawling" or other types of discomfort sensations in the legs?

• Feel a demanding need to move the legs or body to relieve the sensations?

• Are the most notable onsets of RLS at night and evening?

• Do symptoms of RLS worsen in sitting or lying positions?

• Does the patient get at least partial and temporary relief by activity, i.e., walking, leg stretching, leg bending, etc.?

Leg sensations typically occur while sitting down to watch TV in the evening or while lying down trying to go to sleep at night, but they also may occur during the day while trying to nap or while sitting at a desk. Many RLS patients find riding in a car, or other modes of transportation requiring periods of uninterrupted sitting, so troublesome that the need to stand or walk around to relieve the sensations becomes overwhelming.

These questions seem simple to those who have gone from one treatment to another trying to find an explanation for their inability to sleep. They ask, Why has the medical world not been made aware of this disorder that can ruin lives socially, mentally, and physically? Why have victims been forced to accept verbal abuse from physicians, family, and friends with such terms as "hypochondriac," "manic-depressive," "stress," "deep buried secrets," "allergies," "muscle tautness," "leg cramps," "mind over matter," "imaginary ills made up to get attention"?

RLS is so obscure some of the doctors, who are trusted to care for patients, laugh at the name – and unfortunately it does carry a seemingly frivolous title. Perhaps Dr. Ekbom would have done a favor for thousands of sufferers by calling his works by unpronounceable Latin terminology. Then medical students might have studied the syndrome. But this is not the time to bemoan what might have been. Now the truth is out. Let the whole world know there is a physical disorder named RESTLESS LEGS SYNDROME that is treatable. That is step one.

Step two is more difficult. The finding of the proper medication to alleviate the symptoms is not easy. Each patient seems to respond differently. No panacea exists. The patient must find a physician who will take the time to listen and to try appropriate drug therapy.

Dr. Walters lists some of medications which have been tested and proved to be helpful in treating RLS patients:

L-DOPA and carbidopa combination: Sinemet (various strengths including Sinemet CR- time released)

Opioids (Darvon, Percocet, Tylenol with Codeine)

Benzodiazepines (Klonopin, Valium)

Clonidine (Catapres)

Carbamazepine (Tegretol)

Baclofen (Lioresal)

Bromocriptine (Parlodel)

Pergolide (Permax)

Gabapentin (Neurontin)

****All of the above medications must be prescribed by a physician. Patients should be checked to rule out peripheral neuropathy or nerve damage to the legs.

Conversely, some medications may work completely 180° off the recognized use of a drug and sometimes seem to aggravate the condition: some "over-the-counter" sleep inducers may indeed make the restlessness increase, and some medications normally prescribed to calm a patient may actually increase the restlessness. Well-meaning physicians, not understanding the seemingly up-side-down reactions to medication that many RLS patients experience, may endlessly continue the search by trying one useless and sometimes intolerable curative measure after another. Most night walkers have flushed away bottle after bottle of distress-causing pills. In addition to the great financial loss of discarded medication, the sometimes violent reactions cost the patient hours of misery that need not be.

It is true however, that some RLS diagnoses may be more complex because the thief's family includes a number of sleep disturbing disorders which may interact with the syndrome to increase the mystery of proper medication. Then a sleep specialist should be consulted.

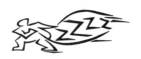

Chapter Four

Myoclonus, the Sleep Thief's Cousin

by Virginia N. Wilson

The sleep thief has many relatives, similar but different. The first cousin which is often associated with and/or confused with restless legs syndrome is nocturnal myoclonus[1], known as Periodic Limb Movements in Sleep (PLMS). These jerking movements recur every twenty seconds during a part of the night's sleep. They may or may not awaken the sufferer. Most patients with RLS have PLMS, but PLMS may occur by themselves in non-RLS patients as well. Patients suffering from the sensations of aching and crawling (paresthesias) while trying to prepare for a night's rest, also, sometimes experience PLMS-like jerking movements while wide awake. These may keep them from falling asleep. The PLMS movements during sleep are not really any different from the PLMS-like jerking movements while

---

[1] Myoclonus is defined as a sudden, brief, shock-like involuntary movement caused by active muscular contractions.

wide awake.   In wakefulness these movements are often less noticeable because the patient moves to suppress them.

Dr. Ralph Pascualy[2] remarked:

> The persons with restless legs have two things they'll suffer from: insomnia, meaning the inability to get to sleep to begin with, and once asleep, the sleep may be easily disturbed.

PLMS may be so gentle the patients may sleep through the night but some PLMS patients may kick very violently and may injure their bed partners or themselves. The spouse of the PLMS patient is sometimes a victim of insomnia as often he or she will be awakened by the partner's incessant kicking. Other parts of the body, especially the arms in addition to the legs, may be involved. The RLS sufferer is usually able to relate to the physician his or her inability to sleep but often it is the spouse of a PLMS patient who reports the violent kicking movements (PLMS) experienced during the patient's sleep.

My husband suffers almost as much as I because of the spasms in my legs. Once I get to sleep, I don't wake up but the spasms continue, and my legs will actually jump off the bed and rise up into the air as if I'm doing leg lifts. This has caused MANY, many sleepless nights for my husband, or I wake up and he is on the couch.

C. L. Wyoming, Michigan

My restless legs are more of a problem for my wife of 31 years. We have a king size water bed and when I am having a restless night and keep flip-flopping, I seriously deprive my wife of her much needed sleep. I can toss and turn all the night and sleep right through it.

R. M., Cromwell, Connecticut

---

[2] See Section I, Chapter 3

Dr. Pascualy also said,

When a person with PLMS goes to sleep the legs keep moving. The person with this problem twitches with a rhythm so the legs may jerk, one or both, and the arms may jerk as well.

But sometimes the leg kicking is so frequent and powerful that the person, even though seemingly asleep is unrested in the morning. So what the patient might say is, 'I couldn't get to sleep for an hour because my legs drove me crazy. Then I slept for six hours and I woke up beat. How could I be so tired since I slept?' Well, this leg movement at night, this myoclonic twitching, is disturbing the brain just a little bit. The brain is disturbed, but not enough to wake up and know there is a problem.

Dr. Pascualy believes that RLS and PLMS together are the primary diagnoses in 13.3% of patients complaining of insomnia and in 6.9% of patients complaining of excessive daytime sleepiness (EDS).

Dr. Bruce Ehrenberg[3] states in the October 1994 *Night Walker* newsletter: Although RLS is fairly common, PLMS actually encompasses a larger group since it includes nearly everyone with RLS, plus a large number of other individuals with only nocturnal movements. Most of these people are not aware of having any leg restlessness during the day or evening, and only come to medical attention because of some other complaint, usually daytime sleepiness caused by the disturbed sleep. Indeed, these patients tend to have more disrupted sleep than the average RLS patient.

[However, this could be just a statistical aberration since PLMS is diagnosed only when a person has a certain number of events during their all-night sleep study, while the diagnosis of RLS does not require a sleep study at all, and many RLS patients have only minimal evidence of leg movements when a sleep study is done.]

---

[3] Bruce Ehrenberg, M.D., New England Medical Center, Tufts University Medical School of Medicine.

"It may be that there are many "normal" people who are having PLMS at night and are totally unaware of it, especially if the leg movements are not strong or if there is no bed partner who is being kicked hard enough to be awakened! We also do not yet know if the patients with PLMS are in any way genetically related to the people with RLS. However, it is true that the same medications tend to be helpful for each group albeit not always with equal benefit (this may be due to the different symptoms being tested: daytime sleepiness for PLMS and leg irritability for RLS).

The Relationship of Restless Legs Syndrome and Periodic Leg Movements in Sleep

David Buchholz, M.D.

Nearly all individuals who suffer from restless legs syndrome (RLS) have periodic leg movements in sleep (PLMS). These movements are typically flexions of the ankle, knee, and/or hip of one or both legs. The movements take up to several seconds each and tend to recur approximately every 30 seconds or so throughout long intervals during sleep.

Although nearly all individuals with RLS also have PLMS, there are many people who have PLMS who do not have RLS. In other words, PLMS is associated with a variety of conditions, only one of which is RLS. People with PLMS may suffer from insomnia as a result of awakening in response to their leg jerks, although they may not realize that leg jerks are the cause of their awakenings. Because of sleep disruption, PLMS can also cause excessive wake time sleepiness. In addition, PLMS disturb the bed partner, often necessitating that he or she sleep in a separate bed. Needless to say, this can contribute to disturbances in relationships between partners.

In attempting to understand the causes of PLMS associated with not only RLS, but also other underlying conditions, several approaches are helpful. To begin with, PLMS bear a strong resemblance to a phenomenon known as the triple-flexion or Babinski response. This is a reflex that is most easily triggered by mechanically stimulating the lateral aspect of the sole of the foot. The reflex is normally present in infants, but disappears around the time that a toddler begins to walk. Reappearance of the reflex later in life is usually associated with an abnormality of the central nervous system (the brain and/or spinal cord) resulting in a loss of the brain's normal inhibition of the reflex. In other words, eliciting a triple-flexion response (flexion of the ankle, knee, or hip) or Babinski sign (flexion of the great toe) during a neurological examination suggests that the patient has some sort of abnormality involving the brain and/or spinal cord.

It turns out that, even though this reflex is normally inhibited by the brain during wakefulness, it is present in normal individuals during non-REM sleep (i.e., the quiet state of sleep during which we do not dream and which comprises most of our sleep time). Moreover, PLMS tends to occur selectively during non-REM sleep.

So far we have established that the movements of PLMS and of the triple-flexion response appear similar and that both phenomena tend to occur during non-REM sleep. Two questions remain: (1) How do RLS and other underlying conditions trigger PLMS? and (2) If PLMS are triple-flexion responses, why do they recur periodically throughout the night?

The sensory input that is required to trigger a triple-flexion response or Babinski sign is characteristically mechanical stimulation of the lateral aspect of the sole of the foot, but other sensory stimuli may be sufficient. In a sense, RLS is a sensory disorder (i.e., causing unpleasant sensations in the legs). The other conditions besides RLS that are associated with PLMS have a common theme of sensory disturbance or abnormal sensory input, including peripheral nerve disorder, compression of lumbosacral nerve roots (sciatica,) circulatory disturbances, and exposure to cold. Other conditions that underlie PLMS may contribute by lowering the threshold for triggering of the triple-flexion response. Examples include medication (such as spinal anesthetic agents), metabolic disturbances, and aging. In other words, RLS and other conditions may predispose to PLMS by providing sensory input capable of triggering the triple-flexion response or by lowering the threshold for activation of the reflex.

The periodicity of PLMS may be explained in two ways. One is that there may be a pacemaker that governs PLMS, analogous to other pacemakers that cycle approximately every 30 seconds or so and govern functions such as heart rate, blood pressure, and respiratory rate. Or, the nerve cells that generate PLMS may have a built-in refractory period; i.e., the nerve cells exhaust themselves temporarily after firing and then require about 30 seconds to recharge and become capable of firing again.

In summary, PLMS may represent periodic occurrence of the triple-flexion response, to which we are naturally predisposed during non-REM sleep. The association of PLMS and RLS, as well as other disorders, may be attributable to sensory disturbance involving the legs or lowering of the threshold for activation of the triple-flexion response. The periodicity of PLMS could be due to a pacemaker with a cycle length of about 30 seconds or a refractory period of the PLMS generator. It is important to recognize that the medications that are useful for RLS (dopamine agonists and opiates) diminish PLMS, and ultimately a better understanding of the mechanism of action of these drugs in RLS and PLMS may lead us to a better understanding of the relationship of these two disorders.

David Buchholz, M.D.
Department of Neurology
Director of Outpatient Services
Johns Hopkins
Baltimore, Maryland

Chapter Five

Other Relatives of the Sleep Thief

by J. Steven Poceta, M.D.

Certain medical conditions can worsen restless legs syndrome, or even be the primary cause of the syndrome. There is likely to be a spectrum in the tendency to have the symptoms of RLS. Of course, certain patients are affected throughout much of their lives and there is little or no influence from their medical status. In other patients, a predisposition to RLS may exist, and under the influence of a medical condition (for example, pregnancy), the symptoms of RLS occur. When the condition is no longer present, the RLS may disappear. In yet other patients, RLS seems to be caused by a specific, perhaps more severe, medical illness, which if alleviated also alleviates the RLS.

Medical research which might allow definitive statements regarding the influence of medical status is lacking. Some of the better-accepted conditions which can cause or exacerbate RLS are:

- Neurologic disorders
- Iron deficiency anemia and gastric resection
- Uremia
- Medications
- Other medical conditions

Neurologic disorders

RLS is ultimately mediated by the central nervous system. It may not be surprising, then, that many neurologic diseases can influence RLS.

Peripheral neuropathy is a dysfunction of some or all of the nerves in the body. The dysfunction is located somewhere between the origin of the nerves in the spinal cord and their termination in muscle and skin in the arms, legs, and trunk. Symptoms of neuropathy usually are tingling, numbness, or weakness starting in the feet or hands, and gradually spreading toward the trunk. Sometimes neuropathies are painful, especially at night, and the unpleasant sensations of neuropathy can be mistaken for RLS. However, it is also true that peripheral neuropathy can cause RLS or make RLS worse. There are many causes of peripheral neuropathy, including diabetes, excessive alcohol intake, amyloidosis, and certain medications such as anti-cancer chemotherapy. Patients with diabetes in particular might have an incidence of RLS as high as 17%. As mentioned, peripheral neuropathy seems to provoke symptoms of RLS in certain individuals. Also, there is some evidence that RLS might be caused by neuropathy too subtle to be detected by clinical evaluation. Usually, treatment specific to RLS is needed. However, in the case of RLS associated with peripheral neuropathy, the medications that treat the pain of neuropathy, for example amitriptyline, might help the RLS somewhat by decreasing pain, but the periodic leg movements in sleep (PLMS) may be made worse. Medications such as L-DOPA are generally useless in neuropathic pain. Because most neuropathies are not easily treated or cured, the exact relationship between them and RLS remains obscure.

Dysfunction at the level of the lower spinal nerve roots in the back seems to cause RLS. Certainly, it is common clinical experience that low back pain and <u>lumbar radiculopathy</u> such as from a bulging disc are associated with RLS. In this situation, the RLS might be felt in the same leg as the sciatica. It is sometimes noticed that patients are cured of their RLS after proper treatment of their back pain, such as with physical therapy or orthopedic surgery. Myelopathy is a spinal cord condition in which the level of dysfunction is in the cervical (neck) or thoracic (back) region, and which causes weakness, numbness, or spasticity. Myelopathy can be caused by discs, viruses, degenerative states, or multiple sclerosis, and might be capable of producing RLS.

Conditions caused by dysfunction within the brain are sometimes associated with RLS. Parkinson's Disease (PD) may be the best example. PD is in large part caused by degeneration of dopamine producing neurons in the substantia nigra nucleus of the midbrain, and is characterized by muscle stiffness, slowness, and tremor. There appears to be a very high incidence of periodic legs movements of sleep (PLMS) in patients with PD. Restless legs have been described in many patients during times in which the dopamine levels are low, such as during so-called "off" spells. However, there is no evidence that RLS can lead to Parkinson's Disease.

Iron deficiency anemia and gastric resection

Dr. Karl Ekbom described a series of patients who had undergone gastric resection, and found RLS in over 11%. He attributed this to malabsorption of certain nutrients. Other researchers have noticed that iron deficiency anemia is particularly likely to produce RLS. In one group of elderly patients, RLS was more common in those who had blood markers of iron deficiency than in those who did not.

I have recently described a case of a 43-year-old man who developed severe RLS over a period of about two years. He had undergone a gastric stapling procedure for obesity several years previously. Otherwise he was in good health, and he took regular injections of B-12 to prevent B-12 deficiency. He described his body near the time of sleep as "full of an energy boom," such that he could not sit still. His wife had noticed prominent jerking of the legs and trunk during sleep. A sleep study showed over 600 strong contractions of leg muscles (PLMS) and very poor sleep. He had only a fair response to temazepam and to propoxyphene. He was then found to be severely iron deficient and anemic, and oral iron replacement was begun. When he did not respond to this therapy, intravenous iron was administered, and the anemia improved. Four months later the RLS was gone, and he was able to sleep without sedatives or medications of any kind. A repeat sleep study showed less than 100 leg movements which were weak and did not disturb his sleep. This case was a convincing example of RLS produced by iron-deficiency anemia in a patient with no known susceptibility. The mechanism is unknown, but RLS could be caused by an iron-dependent mechanism within the brain, such as in the basal ganglia, or perhaps by a peripheral factor such as the reduced oxygen carrying capacity of the anemic blood.

Uremia

Uremia is a term used to connote a high level of blood urea nitrogen, a substance cleared by the kidney, which accumulates in patients with failure of the kidneys (renal failure). PLMS seems to be very common in patients with renal failure, and RLS may occur in 20%. Again the mechanism is unknown, and patients with renal failure have many other metabolic problems or neurological problems, for example anemia or peripheral neuropathy. Nonetheless, this condition is widely recognized to cause or exacerbate RLS, PLMS, and poor sleep, and is usually considered by a physician evaluating RLS.

Medications

Certain medications are recognized occasionally to cause or worsen leg movements (PLMS), but not necessarily RLS. Examples include many of the tricyclic antidepressants, although some of these drugs such as imipramine have occasionally been noticed to help PLMS. In addition, the selective serotonin re-uptake inhibitors such as fluoxetine may produce an increase in PLMS. Many of the neuroleptic agents such as thorazine and haloperidol can produce a restlessness (akathisia) which is similar to, but not the same as, RLS.

Other medical conditions

Orthopedic surgery on the hips and knees seems capable of making RLS worse in susceptible individuals. Some patients notice RLS for the first time during the recovery period from surgery, or notice that their RLS becomes more severe at this time. R. S. was a 67-year-old man who had occasionally had poor sleep associated with a mild feeling of restlessness in both legs. Sometimes at night he would have to walk about, but the problem was not so bad that he ever sought medical help. Unfortunately, shortly after his left total knee replacement, he developed a focal area of restlessness behind the left knee. This feeling was similar to his previous restless feeling, but more severe. It was present primarily at night, and he was up and about most of the night, unable to sleep. L-DOPA (Sinemet) has been effective, but the problem persists over two years.

Even cardiac disease seems capable of worsening restless legs syndrome. A. R. was a 67-year-old woman who had had one and two month bouts of RLS over the course of her life, usually limited to periods of stress or her three pregnancies. However, she came to my attention complaining of severe restlessness at night, such that she was trying to sleep while standing up in the corner or while kneeling at the bedside. Clonazepam and Sinemet were only slightly helpful, and she was quite distraught. Two years previously she had undergone a mitral valve replacement for complications of rheumatic fever. The examination showed right heart failure and diminished mental faculties, and a sleep study showed severe PLMS, restlessness, and periodic breathing (Cheyne-Stokes respiration). She was admitted to the hospital and treated with diuresis, oxygen, and sedatives. Sinemet was continued but eventually changed to pergolide. As her cardiac condition improved, her sleep improved and the severe feeling of restlessness diminished. A later sleep study showed improvement in respiration, PLMS, and sleep quality. She can sleep in her bed, and her alertness and mentation have improved.

In summary, a wide variety of medical conditions can cause or influence RLS, and the best recognized are peripheral neuropathy, lumbar radiculopathy, iron-deficiency anemia, and uremia. In addition, it seems likely that any condition that worsens sleep might worsen RLS. Specific medical conditions need to be considered in any patient with RLS.

J. Steven Poceta, M.D.
Neurologist
Scripps Clinic and Sleep Disorder Center
La Jolla, California

Chapter Six

Sleep Apnea and Narcolepsy

by Virginia N. Wilson

Sleep apnea[1] and narcolepsy[2] have been explored and treated by sleep disorders centers for years since the primary movers of such centers have been physicians treating pulmonary patients. Historically RLS has not been on the agendas of most of these centers, since apnea and narcolepsy are not closely related to restless legs syndrome. Since the lack of sleep is the binding tie of the three, the need for more study and aid for RLS patients has been embraced. Recognition has been long and slow in coming, but now it is considered one of the major causes of sleep deprivation. Also studies

---

[1] Apnea: temporary absence or cessation of breathing. *American Heritage College Dictionary,* 1993.

[2] Narcolepsy: a disorder characterized by sudden and uncontrollable, though often brief attacks of deep sleep, sometimes accompanied by paralysis and hallucinations. Ibid.

may prove that RLS may or may not affect patients with other sleep difficulties.

The following is part of Dr. Pascualy's[3] lecture, designed to help the reader understand and recognize the differences between RLS and these two major sleep disorders.

With sleep apnea the key symptom is snoring. The airway collapses and you stop breathing. You lose oxygen and your brain will awaken. So you have an illness that causes two major kinds of problems. One is that the loss of oxygen affects your heart and your blood pressure and therefore can lead to damage to the cardiovascular system, and the fact that your brain has to awaken to breathe leads to a loss of alertness, tiredness, change in personality, trouble functioning, and perhaps waking. Of course, then there are problems in the marital relationship. Due to the terrible snoring the spouse is disturbed and unable to rest.

Narcolepsy is often confused with apnea in people who are not knowledgeable because both groups are quite sleepy. But in narcolepsy the problem is an inborn error. The person is born with a neurological tendency to not be able to stay awake and therefore may not only have trouble staying awake but they may also suffer from insomnia and can't sleep well either. Most of us might think narcolepsy would mean you just sleep great, you sleep too much, and you fall asleep in your soup, but many people with narcolepsy aren't like that. They're miserably sleepy but they don't fall asleep all the time, they don't sleep well, so they may appear to be insomniacs, which is another kind of problem. They may have very troublesome symptoms when they might feel paralyzed upon awakening and be unable to move. They might have hallucinations which just represent dreams during wakefulness that are very frightening and very distressing; also they may lose their muscle tone if they laugh or are happy or are startled, they might buckle down to the floor or simply feel so weak they can't respond and they take

---

[3] See Section I, Chapter Three

on an odd look. Their faces might droop. Again, socially this is a very problematic kind of experience.

There are about 88 different kinds of disorders that afflict people in their sleep and these two major disorders (apnea and narcolepsy) are important to be familiar with, but there may be more people with various degrees of restless legs than any of the other sleep disorders. In other words, RLS may be possibly the most common of the neurological sleep disorders, more common than narcolepsy certainly, and if we believe that one to three per cent of the population has sleep apnea, perhaps at least that many people have restless legs. And as the population ages, more and more people will develop its (RLS) symptoms.

So these disorders (restless legs, myoclonus, sleep apnea, and narcolepsy) are public health problems. If you have these illnesses you are likely to be at risk while driving and while working, because you are not attentive, endangering other people's well-being not just your own health.

The Good, The Bad and the Restless . . . Plus the Ugly

Lawrence Scrima, Ph.D.

THE GOOD

Why is sleep important? To understand sleep disorders, it is best to know a little about normal, good sleep. Sleep is divided into two types: non-dream sleep and dream sleep. Non-dream sleep, also known as non-REM (rapid eye movement) sleep, has brainwaves that get progressively slower and with higher amplitude, as one goes from light stages one and two sleep to deep stages three and four sleep. Dream sleep, also known as REM sleep or fast brainwave sleep has brainwaves that are similar to awake or stages one and two sleep.

Non-dream sleep has four stages, stages one and two are considered to be light sleep with three and four considered to be deep sleep, since it is easier to awaken someone from light sleep than deep sleep. Sleep changes with age. Infants have about a 90 minute sleep-wake cycle, that is, every 90 minutes they have both sleep and awake periods. Gradually (all too gradual for parents!), the length of both sleep and awake periods increases, so that by school-age, most children are sleeping through the night with only a few requiring a nap during the day. Infants' total sleep time gradually decreases from about 16 hours per day to about 10-12 hours in young school age children, to about 8 hours in young adults, to about 5-7 hours a day in senior citizens. Therefore, sleep, and in particular deep sleep, decreases throughout the life span.

Dream sleep decreases from about 50% in infants to 20%-25% in school age children, remaining at that percentage throughout the life span (if there are no sleep disorders that disrupt dream sleep.)

Growth hormone is released during deep sleep in larger amounts than any other time during the 24 hour day. Growth hormone is important for stimulating growth in children and probably also is important for maximizing healing and renewal of our bodies by production of biochemicals and specialized tissue, such as muscle, skin, red and white blood cells, etc. in adults.

Sleep has been proved to be vital. Animals that are totally sleep deprived die. Even animals that are only REM-sleep deprived die. People who are deprived of sleep, even by reducing their total sleep time by several hours a night, become increasingly uncomfortable; develop diffuse aches and pains; lose energy, motivation, and ability to concentrate; have sensory and cognitive problems, increased mood swings from depression to mania; and in extreme deprivation studies, become very psychologically disturbed, suffering hallucinations, delusions and paranoia.

Sleep also has been proved to be important for learning and memory. Research has shown that memory of information, learned before bedtime, is better in the morning than if information is learned in the morning and tested in the late afternoon. Moreover, my dissertation research, conducted at York University and Sunnybrook Hospital, Toronto, 1979, demonstrated that dream sleep improves memory more than non-dream sleep and that non-dream sleep improves memory more than an equal period of wakefulness (*Scrima*, 1982).

Sleep therefore is vital and essential for physical and mental health, learning and memory, as well as for appropriate adaptive behavior.

THE BAD

Conditions that cause frequent disturbances during sleep cause chronic insomnia and eventually sleep deprivation, as well as excessive daytime sleepiness (EDS). Many conditions can cause frequent disturbances during sleep, such as breathing problems, periodic limb movements syndrome (PLMS, also called nocturnal myoclonus), restless legs syndrome (RLS) with or without PLMS, fragmentary myoclonus, chronic pain, sleep seizures, narcolepsy, and many others.

Sleep apnea (to stop breathing during sleep, in adults: for 10 seconds or longer and in children: depending on the size, a shorter interval) and snoring are breathing problems that typically occur during light sleep and dream sleep. Apnea and snoring can cause insomnia and EDS symptoms by promoting frequent arousals and deprivation of deep sleep and dream sleep.

Narcolepsy is a neurologic disorder that is associated with excessive sleepiness and sudden weakness (cataplexy) when experiencing strong emotions (for example, when laughing, angry, surprised, doing competitive athletics). It is associated with frequent arousals during sleep, and inability to maintain sleep, as well as an inability to remain awake for normal lengths of time, due to what is thought to be a breakdown in the sleep-wake mechanism of the brain (Scrima, 1981). FDA sponsored research I designed, conducted, and reported strongly demonstrated that an investigational biochemical is effective in treating cataplexy and improving excessive sleepiness, without causing any major side effects or habituation (*Scrima,* 1989), (Scrima,1990), (Scrima, 1992). In February of 1995 I began testing a new investigational stimulant for treating narcolepsy that looks promising, based on the double-blind results obtained thus far.

AND THE RESTLESS . . . Plus the Ugly

Can you have RLS and other sleep disorders? Other abnormal conditions occur during sleep, like breathing problems, narcolepsy, chronic pain, and sleep seizures can also cause chronic insomnia and/or EDS. Patients with periodic limb movements in sleep, also called nocturnal myoclonus, can have other sleep disorders. A thorough evaluation by a board-certified sleep disorders specialist is recommended to fully determine if there are one or more of these sleep disorders. Both M.D.s and Ph.D.s can be board-certified by the American Board of Sleep Medicine (ABSM, formerly called A.C P. or Accredited Clinical Polysomnographer), and are qualified to evaluate, test, interpret tests, diagnose, and recommend appropriate treatment options for all sleep disorders.

Patients with sleep apnea or snoring frequently seem to have nocturnal myoclonus. Between 1985 and 1990 I designed and conducted a study for the National Institute of Health (NIH) at the University of Arkansas for Medical Sciences, assessing risk factors of sleep apnea. My colleagues and I found that many males between the ages of 50 and 70 had nocturnal myoclonus without knowing it. Nocturnal myoclonus was much less common among males between the ages of 30 and 50. Sleep apnea can often cause muscle twitches that some patients cease having when sleep apnea is successfully treated. Other patients continue to have muscle twitches even after successful treatment of sleep apnea.

Among several possible reasons why it is not uncommon to see both sleep apnea and nocturnal myoclonus in patients, are two that I favor. If myoclonus develops first, it may eventually promote excessive sleepiness which causes the patient to become less active and gain weight. Being over-weight can cause or exacerbate obstructive sleep apnea, as documented by my NIH study, where essentially all the males 20% or more overweight had obstructive sleep apnea, typically without realizing it (Scrima, 1990). Hence the result is two sleep problems. In such a scenario, successful treatment of sleep apnea would not stop myoclonus from occurring.

Another scenario is that the effort expended to breathe during sleep apnea and snoring may cause rhythmic movements that can look like myoclonus, but these movements are not due to true nocturnal myoclonus and disappear when obstructive sleep apnea is successfully treated.

Some patients with narcolepsy have severe nocturnal myoclonus. I supervised a Ph.D. dissertation research study, designed and conducted by Paul Hartman at the University of Miami in the mid 1980s (Hartman, 1986). Dr. Hartman and I assessed the frequency of nocturnal myoclonus in a consecutive patient series, consisting of 9 patients with only nocturnal myoclonus, as well as in 9 patients with a primary diagnosis of narcolepsy and in 42 patients with the primary diagnosis of sleep apnea. We assessed severity of myoclonus based on the frequency of events and the number of arousals caused by the myoclonus events. The study revealed that many patients with narcolepsy, who also had myoclonus, had more myoclonic induced arousals than patients with the primary diagnosis of only nocturnal myoclonus. One interpretation of this dissertation data is that, for some patients with severe chronic myoclonus, they may become so sleep deprived that they damage the sleep-wake mechanism in the brain and end up with narcolepsy. If this is the case, then early identification of those with nocturnal myoclonus is important. If the sleep of myoclonus patients can be protected by preventing them, then the debilitating effects of this condition could be lessened and perhaps the development of narcolepsy, in severe myoclonus cases, avoided.

Besides genetic factors, there are sleep depriving stress factors that are commonly found in narcolepsy patients' histories, involving irregular sleep-wake schedules, such as due to shift work, or poor sleep quality due to disturbances occurring during sleep, e.g., nocturnal myoclonus and PLMD.

I believe it is important to educate industry and workers about sleep disorders to decrease medical costs due to job and driving accidents, worker burn-out and turn-over rates, as well as to improve job satisfaction, sleep hygiene, workers well being and industry productivity.

ADVICE TO THE RESTLESS

General: Go to bed at about the same time every evening and get up at the same time every morning, allowing for about 7-8 hours of sleep a night. Daily exercise is also very helpful.

Special: For patients with RLS or PLMS, it is important to exercise frequently, perhaps as much as 2 or 3 times a day. Exercise that involves stretching and maximum use of the legs is best, such as walking, swimming, dancing. A hot bath before bed can help relax muscles, as can some leg stretches before bed. If RLS or tightness in the legs recurs during the night, leg stretches can be repeated. It is important to not stay in bed if you cannot achieve sleep within 20-30 minutes, as this can begin to associate the bed and bedroom with not sleeping, worrying, problem solving, and becoming frustrated. Some patients get cold arms and legs during the night, which might also promote muscle twitches. Those patients have reported that wearing socks to bed may be of some benefit.

Can RLS or PLMS be treated? Yes! There are various treatment options available to patients, both prescription and non-prescription, that have been reported to be effective. Most patients can derive at least some relief from symptoms with these remedies.

In a survey I conducted at a hospital for recovering alcoholics, many responders reported that they had RLS-like symptoms and drank alcohol in the evening, at least in part, to get to sleep! Although alcohol can sedate a patient with RLS or PLMS sufficiently to help them get to sleep (Scrima, 1986), alcohol's protective effects only last for about 2-3 hours, after which it causes more sleep disruptions from several side effects. Moreover, alcohol abuse may be one of several possible causes of RLS and/or PLMS. I have some promising research data using a natural substance that so far appears therapeutic and without any major side effects. Further research funding is being sought from public and private sources to further evaluate this potential new treatment. Certainly, more research on causes, additional treatment options, and any potential cure is necessary.

I would like to hear from all patients who have used alcohol to get to sleep and who have any form of nocturnal myclonus. I would also like to hear from all patients who did not notice RLS or nocturnal myoclonus, until they became habitual alcohol drinkers.

RECOMMENDATIONS

If you have chronic insomnia or excessive sleepiness, an evaluation by a board-certified sleep specialist is important to have all possible causes of your symptoms reviewed. An overnight sleep test that includes monitoring your leg muscle activity is also recommended to assess or rule out nocturnal myoclonus, as well as other possible sleep disorders. Sleep tests must be interpreted by a board-certified sleep specialist to obtain the best differential diagnosis consideration. A daytime multiple sleep latency test (MSLT) is also recommended for patients with excessive sleepiness to objectively assess how sleepy they are and to rule out or diagnose narcolepsy. If more than one sleep problem exists, then the patient will need treatment for each sleep problem. Moreover, there must be special consideration for possible adverse drug interactions when multiple treatments are being used.

Lawrence Scrima, Ph.D.
Sleep Alertness Disorder Center
Aurora, Colorado

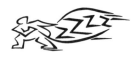

Chapter Seven

RLS: A Family Affair

by Virginia N. Wilson

It has been estimated that one-third of RLS cases are familial: relating to, or characteristic of a family, tending to occur in more members of a family than expected by chance alone, i.e., a disorder. With so many letters coming to us from patients who have positive RLS histories, this family relationship cannot be ignored. Here are a few excerpts. I believe this is one of the most colorful characterizations:

My grandfather had RLS and the family laughed at him for having ants in his pants. He used to have to get out of the car to walk his 'stiff knee' during car trips of a few miles. He was a hoot when traveling from Wilmington to Charlotte. Well, I must have inherited the disease. I've spent thousands trying to find what's wrong with me.

W. H., Dallas, Texas

And this letter rang a loud bell for me:

My mother suffered with restless legs for years. As far as I know she was never treated for it. I did not give it much thought until my legs began to act up, by this time my mother had passed on. I used to sit and rub her legs for her in the nursing home in the last years of her life.

D. J., El Paso, Texas

I'm sure my mother must have suffered with RLS and I did not know. After she came to live with me when she was seventy-five years old, many nights I would hear her crying, praying for relief. I would go in to her room and she would ask me to rub her legs. I have no idea how many tubes of analgesic balm I emptied on her thin legs. Had she too been a victim of RLS and no one understood her agony? Hadn't the doctors treated her regularly for a heart problem and her aching legs that kept her awake at night? We tried one remedy after another often leaving her with uncontrollable legs, confused or weakened so that she could hardly walk. I kept telling her she did not exercise enough. She was not an active athletic woman so the mere word exercise was offensive to her. No 'one - two - three - step - flail - the - air' for her. Foolish stuff! So I suggested that every morning she should take a rag and dust the dining table and chairs, thinking she would be bending, stretching, doing necessary, healthful movements. She looked at me and said, "I didn't come to live with you to do your housework!"

I knew that she had missed the point of my suggestion completely and there were no more remarks about a "daily dozen." At that time I still was convinced that the lack of exercise caused her leg aches, so after I came home from a day's work in our flower shop, I would take her for an evening walk. With her hand clutching my arm for support, she stumbled and lurched along the four blocks of torture – torture for the both of us. I had a suspicion that her inability to control her walking was caused by the strong anti-movement medication the doctor had prescribed. When we stopped that medication, the jerking movements stopped but the leg aches continued. When her condition worsened, she needed around-the-clock care, and we took her to live in a nursing home. Daily she would tell me how she would get up to go to the bathroom and her legs were so weak she couldn't get back in bed so she would kneel there, head resting on the mattress, until a nurse came in. Those were painful days for me, as I felt so very helpless and sorry for her.

I blamed old age for her ills. Some years later, when I was having a particularly bad night, I wrote this poem.

> Mother, I hear you crying
>
> for more liniment and analgesic balm.
>
> Didn't I rub your aching legs
>
> two hours ago?
>
> A virulent cloud of acrid mustard
>
> rising from my tired hands
>
> clears my sinuses and fogs my sight.
>
> I fumble for another tube.
>
> My house reeks of wintergreen.
>
> I look into the mirror.
>
> Tears run down my cheeks.
>
> The voice I'd heard was mine.
>
> My mother died fifteen years ago.

Then I understood. This all happened prior to my own diagnosis of RLS at the sleep center. As I slathered more muscle-relief balm over my quivering legs, I shared the agony she had endured. No more looking for buried secrets in my brain. I had inherited a condition that would cause me pain, similar to hers, for as long as I lived.

Now I am eighty-two years old. I have been on RLS medication for ten years and I'm coping very well. I still think about those nights with my mother and regret that we had no hint that she was suffering from a disorder affecting her legs. Hopefully neither of my children will suffer this confusing and exasperating problem, but time will tell. I have two children. My daughter had polio when she was fifteen and she does not seem to be afflicted with RLS, but she is now suffering from post-polio syndrome. However, recently I was talking with my son, who lives in California, and he mentioned that he is having a time getting to sleep and sometimes it is morning before he finally does doze off. This is not a good sign, but so far he has shown no interest in knowing more about the possible affliction I may have passed on to him. All families have not been so lucky:

I have discovered all of my eleven children have RLS. They are so different physically and emotionally, I find that very interesting. Two of my daughters sleep on the floor when they are really troubled. My granddaughter sleeps on her back with her legs propped up on the wall. None of us sleeps with covers on our legs and we all keep our rooms cold at night.

E. M., Cleves, Ohio.

It [RLS] sure is torture. I have had this all my life, but as I get older it gets worse. All of my children (6) have the same thing and some of my grandchildren.

J. T., Hazel Green, Ala.

Within two years time, my four daughters and I have been afflicted with Restless Legs Syndrome. I find it so strange that five of us would get it within such a short time. Our lifestyles, diets, ages, etc. are quite different. I can find nothing that would account for it happening to all of us within such a short time.

M. A. L., Springville, Utah

Sheila Connolly, Needham, Mass., sent her family records. She and her five siblings (four of them have RLS) and their children have been part of the RLS familial research project since 1990. Sheila was among the original eight letter-exchanging group of RLS victims and it was through her I became acquainted with Dr. Walters. I cannot thank her enough for all her continued support through the years. Last, but certainly not the least, is the reminder to each one about the importance of keeping a family medical record. Research concerning family genes is ongoing. While some of us may not benefit, the hope that something new about RLS will be found to help our children and grandchildren who follow us, is worth any effort we may be called upon to offer.

It's in the Family

Arthur S. Walters, M.D.

and

Bruce Ehrenberg, M.D.

Restless legs syndrome is sometimes inherited. Two separate families with RLS are designated as pedigree #1 and pedigree #2. Each horizontal grouping of the accompanying pedigrees represents a generation. The oldest generations are at the top of the paper and the youngest generations are at the bottom. In the pedigrees, open circles represent women unaffected with RLS, **darkened circles** represent **women affected** with RLS, open squares represent unaffected men and **darkened squares** represent **affected men** (see the accompanying key on the pedigree). A husband and a wife are indicated by a horizontal line joining the middle of a square to the middle of a circle. The children of the marriage are attached by a vertical line to the horizontal line.

RLS follows an autosomal dominant type inheritance pattern. This means that males and females are equally affected and that RLS keeps being passed on from one generation to the next as opposed to an autosomal recessive pattern where a particular genetic disease will skip generations only to return in later generations. Also, only one parent has to be affected with RLS for the children to get it. If RLS runs in your family and you are unaffected with RLS your children will never get it, but the problem is that RLS is often late in onset and, in some cases, it is mild so you can never be sure that you won't pass it on to your children. Notice from the affected pedigrees not all children from parents affected with RLS will get RLS themselves. Sometimes one of four children of a particular parent may get the condition, sometimes three of four may get it. However, statistically it is likely that half of all children of an RLS parent will someday be affected with RLS themselves **if the parent has the inherited form of RLS.**

In pedigree #1, the majority of the cases follow the autosomal dominant pattern, but the case on the far left in the third generation is probably sporadic and not inherited since only one out of 12 children are affected. It is not too unlikely that a sporadic case may occur in an RLS family by chance alone because RLS is very common. A recent Canadian survey suggested that RLS may exist, to varying degrees of severity, in up to 10% to 15% of their population. The good news is that not all RLS is hereditary. The bad news is that between a third to a half of all cases of RLS are of the hereditary type.

We are currently involved in a search for the gene in restless legs syndrome that causes it to be passed on from one generation to the next. As of this writing we have collected blood from over 120 members of seven large families similar to the ones outlined here. To our total of seven families, Dr. Bruce Ehrenberg of Tufts New England Center, Boston, Massachusetts, has contributed two families. Including our own group, Dr. Elio Lugaresi and Dr. Giorgio Coccagna of the University of Bologna, Italy; Dr. Claudia Trenkwalder of the Max Planck Institute for Psychiatry, Munich, Germany; Dr. Dan Picchietti of the Carle Clinic, Urbana, Illinois; and Dr. Mitchell Brin from Mt. Sinai Medical Center, New York City, each has contributed one family.

All of these investigators have given diligently of their time tracking down, interviewing, examining new patients, creating family trees, and, most importantly, drawing blood which is now being processed and analyzed for the culprit gene. It is our sincere hope that the discovery of this gene will lead to new and better therapies for the restless legs syndrome.

Arthur S. Walters, M.D.
Department of Neurology
Robert Wood Johnson Med. School
New Brunswick, New Jersey and VA
Medical Center, Lyons, New Jersey

Bruce L. Ehrenberg, M.D.
Department of Neurology
Tuft University-New
England Medical Center
Boston, Massachusetts

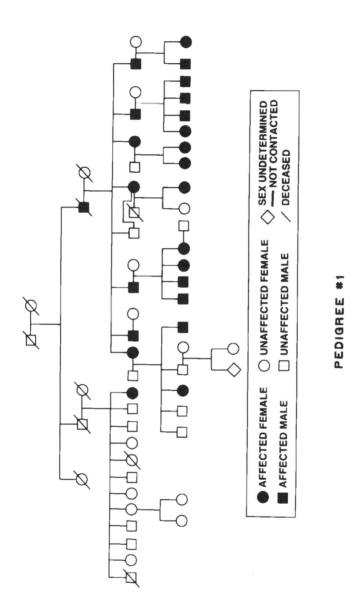

PEDIGREE #1

AFFECTED FEMALE ○ UNAFFECTED FEMALE ◇ SEX UNDETERMINED

■ AFFECTED MALE □ UNAFFECTED MALE — NOT CONTACTED

/ DECEASED

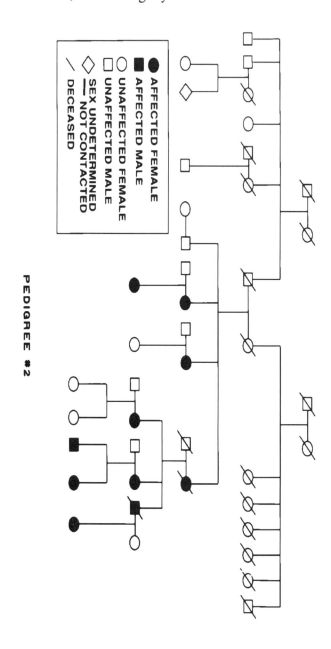

PEDIGREE #2

Chapter Eight

Childhood "Growing Pains"

by Virginia N. Wilson

Until recently the lack of sleep during childhood may not have been a primary concern in the medical world, except perhaps for parents and pediatricians. But now we realize that sleep deprivation is a serious problem for the young as well as for the mature adult. The fact that most RLS victims do not recognize the problems of poor sleep patterns until late in life has left a void in the study of this disorder in childhood. Mothers all know that a tired child is a problem child, cranky and difficult to reason with or even chastise.

Actually the only thing that I remember about my very early childhood was sleeping curled in a fetal position and rocking myself to sleep while I held my legs tightly because of my great fear of having my legs cut off if they happened to stray outside my bed. I must have been very young for I recall that I always felt safe inside the upright slats of my baby bed. I knew that no one in my family would cut off my feet, but I feared some strange creature might steal in the house and do the deed. When I read the comic strip about

Calvin and Hobbes I think that perhaps I dreamed up wild, dangerous creatures during my sleep. I don't know. But I have never entirely forgotten the real terror I experienced then. If I complained of leg aches I was told I was experiencing "growing pains" and that every child had them. I accepted that as a part of growing up.

Sitting quietly has always been a problem for me. As a child I was like a jack-rabbit ready to hop off any moment. Fifteen years ago I chose my present physician, a pediatrician, now a general practitioner, because I heard he did well with hyperactive children. I told him I felt like a little kid whose mother had threatened to spank if I didn't sit still and be quiet, and my answer would have to be, "Spank me, I can't sit still." He prescribed a well-known medication given to hyperactive children. It did help to quiet me. He kept searching for answers to my problem until I was diagnosed with RLS six years later. Since then he and I have explored this disorder together.

I had not thought much about my childhood until I began to read the notes written as letters on the backs of query sheets I had sent out to Night Walkers and the truth struck me very hard: I was a "problem" child in grade school. My lessons came very easily to me and I would finish my reading assignments or papers in a short time. Then I began to bother the slower students around me. Fortunately my teachers all seemed to understand that I had boundless nervous energy which they drained off each day with a myriad of tasks to perform – erasing the blackboards, passing out papers, keeping the library straight, and when I was in the upper grades I was sent to help the teachers in the lower grades.

Many of our Night Walkers experienced the same childhood jittery days and nights. It seems that some started experiencing RLS earlier than others!

At the time of my birth there were rumors about babies being switched in maternity wards. My mother states that she was sure she had the right baby because, as they took me out of her and placed me at her side, I drew up my leg as if it had cramped. As far as I know I have had RLS from that day to this.

J. M., Las Vegas, Nevada

As a child I got my butt hit more than I care to remember and was told, "Stop that damn leg shaking. You're just as jumpy as your pa." Cross your legs and they start twitching like keeping time with music.

Now, I wear a head-set to work at my press. I'm on my feet constantly. When I sit for over 15 to 30 minutes, my leg muscles tighten up and get very painful to touch or massage.

L. H., Tampa, Florida

The first time I can remember having restless legs was when I was in grade school and went to see "Mary Poppins" That was the longest movie I ever sat through.

A. R., Tomball, Texas

I thought back on my childhood and BOOM! this came to mind: crying because the pain was so bad. My mother would lay hot or cold washcloths on my legs until I fell asleep. She called it "growing pains."

J. D., Glendale, California

As a child my legs always bothered me. I could not sit for very long, and I would not be able to go to sleep at night. I could not sit through a movie. When riding on a bus, I had to stand even though there were plenty of seats available. The doctors did not know what it was and I remember them saying that it was just "growing pains!"

The only relief I could get, especially at bedtime was to take hot baths. Even then, I would usually have to get up 1-3 times each night, having to repeat the hot baths so I could go back to sleep. Also I could never put covers on my legs until after I was asleep, if I got cold, I would "cover up." During the day my legs did not bother me as much, but I always had trouble sitting through a movie or a play without wanting to get up and stretch my legs.

I have a son who is 14 years old and a daughter 19 years old. My son, at an early age started to have some of the same symptoms that I had. He called it the "Jiggles" referring to the way his legs felt. He too started to take hot baths in order to go to sleep but I don't think that he gets up in the middle of the night. My daughter says her legs bother her sometimes but I do not think it is anything like I had or possibly my son has.

R. W., Louisville, Kentucky.

I had quite a shock when I went into high school and was sent to detention after school every day for two weeks because I couldn't sit still in study halls. I solved that. I volunteered to help in the library and on the school paper and the year book. I joined the debate team and the dramatic club. Later I was elected to the student council and became an officer in many clubs. I offered my services for anything that let me move about. The teachers loved me. Gladly they received hours of free help. I was a human dynamo for three years. Then, one morning in my senior year, I collapsed in our bathroom, unable to walk. The teachers, the deans, and the principal sent me notes of apology, all blaming themselves for allowing a student to almost work herself to death. After two months of complete bed rest and daily meals of broiled almost-raw liver, goat's milk, and whole-wheat breads, I was able to return to my classes, but school was never the same. The hours of student assistance and the number of outside activities any student could participate in were drastically cut. Those rules still apply at that school today.

I didn't get to go to college because of my weakened condition, but when I retired I continued my education at the University of North Florida in Jacksonville. It was a challenge trying to sit quietly in classes, but I loved every minute of it and made a lot of friends among classmates more my grandson's age than mine. Even though I couldn't sit still, I did a lot of research in bits and spurts and did all my writing on my computer while standing up.

My childhood love of study and my youthful days of activity have always sustained me well. In 1990 I began exchanging letters with eight other RLS victims and when our group began to grow we felt a need for some type of questionnaire to gather information to share.

We theorized that we might stumble on to something valuable to RLS research. And we did, but not from any of the questions asked.

I was amazed at the number of Night Walkers who voluntarily wrote notes on the back of the query sheets saying, "I had trouble with aching legs as a child and my mother said I had 'growing pains.'" I began to watch for these notations. When I had one hundred of them, I told Dr. Walters and sent him the questionnaires. From that unexpected discovery, research began on childhood RLS.

With the help of Dr. Kathleen Hickey, his student aide, Dr. Walters began a comprehensive study of possible childhood RLS. Soon others joined in the search for new areas of childhood sleep deficit problems. Now Attention Deficit Hyperactivity Disorder (ADHD) has come under study. I am pleased to know that our Night Walkers have contributed to helping unravel a puzzling mystery of RLS. Perhaps in the future we will be able to answer the question asked in this letter from a Night Walker who suffers with a serious case of RLS:

Do you know if there might be a relationship [of RLS] with minimal brain dysfunction or learning disabilities? Both of my boys had it - one severe - in 2nd grade he didn't know the right from the left side of the body and it wasn't a popular diagnosis - I had to get information from Boston to find a therapist to work with him and did years of exercises with him. He's typical - above average intelligence but couldn't sit still. Still can't spell but has outgrown the hyperactivity he had as a child. The second boy, the 19-year-old, had it, but milder. I found out that, too, is genetic because their dad had the same problem as a child and was treated in Boston.

S. R., Port St. Lucie, Florida

This and many more questions are awaiting answers from our researchers. "Growing pains" may be a childhood myth but we need information to ensure that future generations will not have to endure the myth.

Growing Pains: RLS in Children

by Daniel Picchietti, M.D.

"Growing Pains" is a term that may turn out to have very special and significant meaning for families of RLS sufferers. Currently, pediatricians think of growing pains as a transient and insignificant problem that children will outgrow. New evidence indicates that some children with growing pains actually have RLS.

Does RLS occur in children? Recently we have found that the answer is an unequivocal, "YES." Letters to the Night Walkers Support Group and a subsequent survey via the Night Walkers were important impetus to the scientific study of childhood RLS. As in adults, RLS in children can be a "silent masquerader" that is often mistaken for other things. However, the misdiagnoses in children are often different than in adults. We have now seen over 100 children with RLS who have presented in a variety of ways: night jerks thought to be seizures, leg pains dismissed as "only growing pains," daytime attention-span problems or hyperactivity brought on by poor sleep, bedtime struggles, frequent sleep-walking, and even severe headaches set off by poor sleep.

In the remainder of this chapter, I would like to outline the development of ideas about childhood RLS. The experience my own family has had with RLS as well as other case histories will be used to illustrate these concepts.

Detective Work

Dr. Walters and I met by chance at a Neurology meeting in Chicago in 1989. He was presenting some preliminary work on the search for the RLS gene, when I mentioned that my wife and other members of her family had RLS. In 1983 I had stumbled across a description of this presumed-unusual problem in a book on rare neurological diseases, which led to a diagnosis of my wife's problem. Her father was diagnosed in 1985, when we found RLS by chance while doing a sleep study for what we thought might be sleep apnea. Her family subsequently agreed to become part of the RLS gene-study group.

On Thanksgiving 1991 I realized that my 4-year-old boy and 22-month-old girl also had RLS. They both fell asleep, exhausted, at a late-night concert. Lying in my lap, both had the characteristic, repetitive leg twitches of RLS. Perhaps not coincidentally, they both had consumed a lot of caffeine that day. At the concert, it became crystal clear to me that 1) The intermittent foot-rubbing, the complaint of leg "owies" at night, and their annoying habit of "playing chase" at bedtime were much more than growing pains or normal childhood behavior and 2) RLS **can** occur in children. They subsequently had sleep studies and became the first two children in the medical literature to have RLS described in detail. That was published in the October 1994 issue of *Pediatric Neurology (Walters, 1994)*.

The next big clue came in 1992 after Dr. Walters and I discussed his presentation at the Sleep Meeting in Phoenix. He and Dr. Hickey wrote up three siblings, then 18-22 years old, who had a possible misdiagnosis of RLS as growing pains and hyperactivity when they were younger. Since I treat children for Attention Deficit-Hyperactivity Disorder (ADHD,) I promised to ask more specific questions about RLS in these children.

ADHD is a problem that affects an estimated 3% to 5% of school-age children. It is characterized by a short attention span. Impulsiveness and a high activity level may also occur. The poor attention span for the child's age is most evident in tasks requiring sustained mental effort and sequential tasks. Getting schoolwork or chores done is often a major struggle. ADHD is not a disease, but a constellation of symptoms, no single one of which is unique, and no combination of which is unique. ADHD has different causes in different children.

Previous reports in medical literature had commented on poor sleep in some ADHD children, but very little had been made of this, including no link to RLS. Realizing that we all have trouble focusing and paying attention when we have had inadequate sleep, Dr. Walters and I wondered if RLS could aggravate or cause ADHD in some children.

We found over 40 children in the next year. Families were thrilled that someone was finally taking their children's sleep problems seriously. We presented 14 of those cases at the Sleep Meeting in Boston in 1994, proposing a link to ADHD. Survey data from the RLS Night Walkers support group was also presented by Dr. Walters indicating that almost 20% of adult RLS sufferers recalled the onset of their symptoms between birth and 10 years of age. Almost 25% more recalled onset between 11 and 20 years of age. These leads were developing into a much bigger and more complete picture.

AGE SPECIFIC MANIFESTATIONS

The following are some actual cases of how RLS may appear in childhood.

Baby Blues

By one year of age, Nicole's parents had figured out how to regulate her sleep patterns. She had never been an easy baby when it came to sleep, but if she had followed in her older brother's footsteps, things would have gotten worse. Nicole's mother, Nanette, was now pregnant with their third child and neither parent could imagine repeating the sleep onset problems and frequent night waking problems they'd had with their first one.

Nanette knew her own RLS would get worse as the pregnancy progressed. Her leg jerks had become quite disruptive to her husband's sleep but when the idea of sleeping in separate beds was first discussed Nanette stated, "If you are going to move to another bed, you might as well move out." She was upset at the suggestion that the assumed marital agreement of couples sleeping together would be broken, but then she remembered how her own mother had been a victim who had endured 30 years of sleeping with a husband who suffered with RLS. Nanette relented and after the couple decided to sleep in different beds she found her husband to be more energetic and helpful. This simple change in parental sleeping arrangements sparked a re-examination of how they dealt with little Nicole's and her brother's sleep.

Nanette and her husband formulated a plan to deal with Nicole's sleep. Using ideas they had developed and ideas in Dr. Ferber's *Solve Your Child's Sleep Problems* book, Nicole's parents set some simple rules. They adhered to a strict and consistent sleep schedule for Nicole. They looked up how long she should sleep for her age and made sure Nicole stayed in her crib that long. Bedtime followed a consistent routine of snack, bath, book, then bed. She was put in bed awake and was never rocked to sleep or given a bottle to fall asleep. If she fussed after being put to bed, her protests were ignored, because by now her parents knew the difference between fussing and a "hurt," "sick," or "hungry" cry. Nighttime arousals were common but also ignored. They never allowed her to sleep in her parent's beds. Fortunately, she did not learn to climb out of her crib. Using this routine, Nicole's sleep pattern and her parents' sleep patterns smoothed out a lot.

Confirmation that RLS was Nicole's underlying problem came later. At 22 months, repetitive leg jerks in sleep were observed by her father. Intermittent rubbing of one foot on another and complaints of leg "owies" at night became evident during her second year. Nicole's parents noted that an irregular sleep schedule and caffeine appeared to aggravate her leg "owies" and sleep disruption, so care was taken to regulate those factors.

We have found that "creepy-crawly" and other unpleasant sensations of RLS are much less prominent in children than in adults. The decrease in sleep **quantity** caused by not getting to bed, and staying in bed, as well as the decrease in sleep **quality** associated with the jerks are much greater problems. Fortunately, forcing the child to stay in bed **decreases** the lower-extremity discomfort after a few nights, as sleep quantity and quality improve. Unless she is off her regular sleep schedule or gets caffeine, Nicole does not complain of leg "owies."

Many parents find ignoring nighttime fussing or crying very hard to do. They are often run down by this time and lack patience. They want to quickly satisfy their child's apparent plea for help to get to sleep. Unfortunately, rocking or sleeping with the child promotes dependence on the parent for sleep onset. A truly "good" parent must set the stage, then stand back and allow the child to struggle a bit to achieve independence.

The Baby From Hell

Gregg is 17 years old and is better on medication for RLS. His parents can now look back and laugh about "the baby from hell." His mother is certain that he never slept through the night until he was 17. As an infant, he had jerks in his sleep like "bolts of electricity," sleeping less than two hours in a stretch. He had "severe colic" during his first year of life which the pediatrician said he would get over. The pediatrician advised that they try buying pint bottles of benadryl and "loading" him with it at bedtime. His leg discomfort was written off as "growing pains." Both of Gregg's parents probably have RLS and he may have inherited a double dose of the RLS gene.

Gregg represents an extremely severe case of RLS, a situation I have seen in three other babies. One had been misdiagnosed as having seizures at night. Two had a good response to a medication called clonazepam at low doses. A family history of RLS was the key to understanding the extreme sleep problem in each case.

Terrible Twos

Matthew had never been a good sleeper, but the situation got worse when he moved from his crib to a regular bed at two-and-one-half years old. Bedtime followed a strict sequential routine, but he would typically reappear for unwanted "curtain calls" after being put to bed. Since the age of two years, he had complained of occasional leg and foot pain at night. He liked to "play chase" just before bed, stating, "My feet just want to move. They want to run." He would rub one foot on the other or wiggle his feet whenever sitting or lying, presumably to relieve the leg dysesthesias. Instituting a "no-out-of-bed" rule helped defuse the struggles, but sleep latency was typically more than fifteen minutes. Nocturnal awakenings were common with frequent attempts to sleep in his parents' bed. His parents banished him from their bed, explaining, "You would allow him to sleep with you, if you like to get head-butted and body-slammed in sleep." Matthew's parents realized that the more tired he was (short of exhaustion) the **harder** he was to get to sleep. So, they almost never let him stay up late, to avoid "paying for it the next day" via irritable and unruly daytime behaviors.

A sleep study on Matthew, when he was five-and-one-half years old, showed twelve lower-extremity jerks per hour. Subsequently it was discovered that caffeine appeared to aggravate his problems. He had more difficulty falling asleep and staying asleep, and was more irritable the next day after he had consumed caffeine. This was true even if only small amounts of caffeine were taken early in the afternoon. When he was put on a caffeine-free diet that excluded chocolate (which contains small amounts of caffeine) his sleep onset and maintenance improved notably the first week. A blinded trial back on caffeine caused deterioration in his sleep as well as reappearance of notable daytime irritability, impulsiveness and hyperactivity over a two week time span.

He is currently in second grade and he self monitors his caffeine intake. He has attention-span problems in school but has responded to structure in his routine, with fair but firm consequences. Matthew's case illustrates two common, probable aggravants of RLS in children: sleep deprivation and caffeine.

Too tired to sleep?

The statement "I am too tired to sleep" is recognized as a contradiction or oxymoron by most good sleepers. Good sleepers find it easier and easier to fall asleep the more tired they are. However, many RLS sufferers recognize that their RLS gets worse as they become more sleep deprived, making sleep **harder** to get, until they reach the point of exhaustion. Unfortunately many parents, RLS sufferers, and doctors misinterpret this "alerting" effect of sleep deprivation as "not needing much sleep." RLS sufferers then try to function while chronically sleep deprived, attributing lack of attention, poor memory, and moodiness to things other than the sleep deprivation.

More research is needed, but caffeine may prove to be an equally important aggravant. It may not be coincidence that the great clinical neurologist, Thomas Willis, first described RLS in 1685, soon after coffee and tea had been introduced into Europe. We have done blinded caffeine trials on three children, all showing sleep deterioration and subsequent daytime irritability with caffeine. Most of my adult patients who abstain from caffeine, note that re-introduction of even small amounts of caffeine will aggravate their RLS and make their medication less effective. Two adults reported that they did not know until the next day that their morning coffee was caffeinated (instead of decaf) and had particularly bad RLS that night.

Why then do some adults claim that caffeine helps their RLS? It may be because the caffeine aggravation is a **delayed** effect, probably due to a caffeine metabolite (a chemical that the body breaks caffeine down into, before getting rid of it). For two to four hours, caffeine acts as a stimulant, alerting a person and thereby reducing the RLS sensations. However, the metabolite may then hang around, and aggravate the RLS, causing worse sleep, which makes the person want more caffeine the next day . . . a vicious cycle. We have provided at this chapter's end, a list of caffeine sources with the admonition: *"Caffeination Without Cognition Is Chaos."*

Since sudden cessation of caffeine can cause withdrawal symptoms (headache, muscle aches, fatigue, etc.), gradual tapering is suggested. Consult your doctor if you have any questions about this. Also, if caffeine's alerting effect is being used to partially suppress severe daytime sleepiness (such as drowsiness at the wheel), then the underlying cause of the sleepiness should be treated, before caffeine is withdrawn.

Ozone Layer

Jumping Jimmy is a 7-year-old second grader who went to the doctor because of school problems. In spite of being gifted, he struggled to work up to his potential in class, particularly with repetitive or monotonous tasks. He was never known to fall asleep in class but he did "zone out." In first grade, the teacher allowed him to put his shirt over his head for a few minutes, after which he seemed better. The second grade teacher found this unacceptable. Jimmy stated, "I hop around to keep myself awake; I do it when I am tired." His teacher rated him as having poor attention span, poor independent work, and hyperactivity as compared to his classmates.

His parents thought he was more easily excited, more irritable, and "crankier" than his siblings. At night he experienced intermittent leg aches, described as "someone trying to pull my legs off," which were thought to be "growing pains." They occurred when he sat or lay and subsided with movement. Massaging the legs helped. He chronically had difficulty falling asleep and staying asleep.

As the doctor asked more specific RLS questions, Jimmy's mother exclaimed, "That must be what I have!" She complained of always being tired. She had typical RLS leg aches experienced on a regular basis. She woke frequently during the night. Her husband complained of her twitching in her sleep, which bothered his sleep. Previous discussion with her physician, brought no specific diagnosis for her "tiredness." Discussion of her childhood revealed a history of "growing pains" and some attention-span problems, but no hyperactivity in school. The father had no symptoms of RLS, but interestingly, had a history indicative of attention-deficit disorder with hyperactivity as a child, which he appeared to have outgrown.

A lengthy discussion of Jimmy's school problems ensued. While he met standard criteria for ADHD, it was proposed that his ADHD **might** be aggravated or caused by RLS. Given the choice of proceeding with a trial on ritalin vs. pursuing the sleep disorder, his parents enthusiastically wanted to look into the sleep issue.

Both Jimmy and his mother had sleep studies which confirmed RLS. With set sleep schedules, caffeine abstinence, and RLS medcation at night, both are functioning much better. Jimmy's teacher describes him as "no longer in the ozone layer" and by rating scales notes a clear-cut improvement in his attention span. He got straight A's on his last report card. His parents note that his sleep has improved, he is calmer, he is less irritable and argues less with his sister. Jimmy's mother feels she can now cope with her parenting duties more effectively, and has been able to provide more structure to his environment.

This case illustrates five points:

• The first is the link between RLS and ADHD. In our original report, Dr. Walters and I found approximately 20% of ADHD children that we studied have evidence for RLS. We think that the poor quality and quantity of sleep in these children causes or aggravates their difficulty with attention span, follow-through, and mood. Poor sleep can cause such daytime problems for anyone. Treatment directed at improving sleep in these RLS children has usually resulted in very positive daytime benefits.

• The second point is that RLS often runs in families as a dominant trait (that means there is a 50-50 chance of an affected parent passing it on to a child).

• Third, the parent, as well as the child, is usually undiagnosed. In 26 cases of RLS children we recently reviewed, no parent had a previously-made diagnosis of their own RLS.

• The fourth is that "dysfunctional family" takes on a whole new meaning if the problem child has a parent with untreated RLS whose restless sleep may be disturbing **both** parent's sleep.

• The fifth point is more complicated. After working with over 100 RLS families, I have the distinct impression that young RLS children do better in homes where the parents have a more autocratic (strict) approach, than a permissive or democratic parenting style. However, this **may** not hold true for RLS teens.

Split Personality

Maggie's mother states that her sixteen-year-old daughter has always had sleep-onset problems and did not sleep through the night until three years old. She has a history of growing pains and occasionally gets "fizzy" feelings in her legs. She has chronically had only six and one half to seven hours' sleep at night. She got by in school, but was an underachiever and typically put things off until the last minute. She had trouble getting motivated and staying organized. While she could be quite charming and engaging in public, she tended to be irritable and moody at home. She had chronic dark circles under her eyes. Recently she had discovered that she could cover the dark circles with cosmetic foundation and was delighted the first day she used this to have several people at church remark how bright and healthy she looked.

After diagnosis and treatment of her RLS with a regular sleep schedule, caffeine abstinence, and nighttime medication, her mother notes that she has a better attitude at home and is not so easily angered. Maggie's grades have improved and she claims to be more alert, to think more clearly, and finds her schoolwork is easier to do.

Maggie's case illustrates the odd duality that some teens and adults with RLS feel. When highly stimulated, motivated, or when "on stage," they realize an ease, vitality, and potential that they find difficult to attain when more relaxed or involved in more routine activities. This can be a source of great personal frustration.

Where to now?

These observations regarding RLS in children are a good start. However, much more work needs to be done to establish a broad scientific foundation for diagnosis and treatment. We need proven methods to sort out this "silent masquerader" from other problems it may mimic.

"Growing pains" may turn out to be an important clue to RLS in childhood. In that sense, "growing pains" has a much broader meaning, encompassing the nighttime and daytime problems that may result in childhood from RLS. We hope that continued work on understanding and ultimately treating this problem during childhood will be as fruitful as these early observations indicate.

Daniel Picchietti, M.D.
Pediatric Neurology Sleep Center
Carle Clinic
Urbana, Illinois

CAFFEINE SOURCES

Food

Sodas/Pop

colas (unless caffeine-free)

Usually caffeine is not in lemon-lime (7-Up, Sprite), root beer, or orange. Regular Mountain Dew does have caffeine (there is a caffeine-free version).

If in doubt whether a soda is caffeine-free, check the list of **ingredients** for the word "caffeine" (the "nutritional information" section is not the place to look).

Tea (brewed and iced)

Decaf tea is not recommended either, since there appears to be some caffeine or related compounds left that can still cause a problem. Caffeine-free herbal tea should be OK.

Coffee

Decaf coffee in morning is probably not a problem, for adults.

Chocolate and Cocoa

These substances contain some caffeine and a relatively large amount of a related compound called theobromine. Make sure children are not getting chocolate milk at school.

Medication

Some pain relievers such as Excedrin

Diet medications such as Dexatrim

Stay awake pills such as No-Doz

Some prescription medication such as Esgic

Substitutes

Caffeine-free sodas are fine (decaf beverages are not; they still have some caffeine).

Carob is a chocolate substitute available in health food stores that does not have caffeine.

Butterscotch morsels and white morsels (Nestle) are good for baking and snacking.

"Caffeination Without Cognition Is Chaos"

Chapter Nine

Being Both the Doctor and the Patient

Frankie Roman, M.D.

Nightwalkers in white lab coats! Given the high prevalence of Restless Legs Syndrome, with victims from all walks of life, it is not surprising that health care professionals are also afflicted. However, in a profession with very little margin for error, the effects of RLS can be devastating!

As a fellow sufferer of RLS, I have "talked the talk, and walked the walk." Besides completely disrupting every sphere of my life, the results were exponential with RLS negatively influencing my career as a medical doctor.

During my medical internship my ignorance directly impacted on patient care. Many a long night on-call, I paced the hospital hallways trying to relieve the burning and aching in my legs. Occasionally, I evaluated patients who described my own symptoms. Little did I realize my own malady was kicking me. I would reassure the patient "he/she had nothing" and if absolutely necessary prescribe Quinamm for the vague and all-encompassing diagnosis of leg cramps. Then,

I would proceed to instruct the nurses not to page me for such a trivial problem and rush back to the house officer's call room to deal with my own restless legs and overall fatigue. It would always take me several days to recover from the strenuous physical activity of a night on-call. Many a day I missed morning report, unable to wake up on time. And, on the days I did make it, I would be confused, irritable, and fatigued. In retrospect, it seemed I was always running, always in a hurry! In this dramatic vacuum I completed my medical training. It was only during my Fellowship in Sleep Disorders Medicine at Scripps Clinic and Research Foundation that I came to the painful reality of my own illness. In my defense, albeit a poor one, I had had absolutely no exposure to sleep disorders during college, medical school, or residency. This total lack of awareness of sleep disorders among doctors is not unusual as documented on a survey of U.S. medical schools by Rosen and colleagues (Rosen et al., 1994). Overall, less than two hours of total teaching time is allocated to sleep topics with thirty-seven medical schools reporting no structured teaching at all. The reasons for this travesty were multifactorial and identified as lack of qualified faculty, no curriculum time allotted for sleep topics, and the need for structured clinical and educational resources. Unfortunately, this bleak environment continues to exist in our educational system. Despite this, each and everyone of us should forsake self-pity and apathy. As with any other chronic illness, education and control are crucial keys to a prosperous and productive life. Physicians must take an unequivocal role of leadership in the management of RLS.

The following is an array of coping strategies ranging from plain common sense to ingenious but unproven remedies. Apply them as need be and, more importantly, add your own to the list.

Rules of Empowerment

(for the physician, lawyer, pastor, teacher, executive, author, TV personality, senator, ambassador, head of state, or ordinary citizen who may be a victim of RLS)

1. Introspection with systemic evaluation of your own health. Understand that many of the identified causes of RLS are infrequent.
2. Study your relatives. Since RLS runs in families, there may be a family member you can help.
3. Review all your medications, as this may be a rare cause of RLS.
4. Specifically for physicians: Although the temptation is great, never self prescribe controlled substances due to impaired-physician issues that may arise.
5. Eliminate coffee and other caffeinated products.
6. Adhere to strict sleep hygiene measures.
7. Sleep in. Historically, the best sleep in patients with RLS occurs in the early morning hours.
8. Flexible work hours with a later start time.
9. Wear slip-on shoes giving you the capability of taking off your shoes easily for relief and stretching.
10. Have an enclosed desk. You then have the ability to stretch and move your legs without being observed.
11. Give patients or other visitors a tour of your office and/or sleep center thereby giving you the opportunity to stretch and walk between each patient evaluation.
12. Specifically for physicians: Share anecdotes with patients. Knowing someone has walked in their shoes is a very comforting sensation to them.
13. Have an outlet for stress - hobbies, sports, etc.
14. When all else fails and you need to get out of a patient's room or meeting, page yourself so you may leave without incident. Most beepers can go off with a flick of a switch.
15. Educate, educate, and educate.

Frankie Roman, M.D.
Director, Center for Sleep Disorders
Massillon, Ohio

SECTION II

The Patient, the Doctor, and Medication

Chapter One

The Pain of Being Misdiagnosed
by Virginia N. Wilson

"Misunderstood" is the word almost every RLS victim uses to describe his or her situation in daily living. The second most used word is "misdiagnosis" while trying to cope with the medical world. The rich and the poor, the young and the old, the strong and the weak, the good and the bad are all equal before the Sleep Thief. Money does not buy an understanding attitude from relatives, friends, or physicians, nor can money buy a cure because the Sleep Thief is not tempted by bribes. He maintains his power by teasing, tickling, pulling, tugging, bashing, and cramping legs, and sometimes arms, until his victims beg for mercy, crying aloud for relief from this mysterious malady.

A neurologist charged me $120 for reading a brain scan that had cost $764 and then found nothing wrong with me. No advice. It is incredible there are so many "specialists" totally unaware of RLS.

S. B., Bozeman, Montana

Doctors think we are just a bunch of "Nervous Nellies."

M. D., Ankeny, Iowa

I have never had a doctor who really knew what to prescribe. One suggested an over-the-counter vitamin, good for poor circulation. Doctors either shrug their shoulders or nod their heads saying, "Yes, I have heard of it." Period.
                                                    L. S., Fredricksburg, Texas

My own experiences parallel those suffered by many RLS patients. For years I sought help for my inability to sleep. All the physicians seemed concerned but not one came near to solving my problem, which worsened year by year. One allergist wrote on his report that I was a hypochondriac. A psychiatrist assured me I had a deeply buried secret that kept my mind from allowing my body to rest. His psychologist colleague enrolled me in his "tell all and wash away" sessions. For weeks, I spent long hours listening to lives broken because of childhood sexual abuse, failed marriages, failed love affairs, failed finances, failed and repentant alcoholics and drug addicts and I kept wondering what I was doing among all these unhappy people who had made messes of their lives. I remained silent. I searched my soul for all the bad things that might have happened to me. There was none. Finally I called a halt.

"Doctor," I said, "I am happy, prosperous, and loved – but sleepless. I get very depressed listening to all these sad, messed up lives. All I want is a good night's sleep." I walked out with a feeling of great relief. I felt very fortunate that I only had a sleep problem to worry about.

I told the psychiatrist that I had found no hidden secrets in my life and he promptly replied, "Then it must be a chemical unbalance causing your problem. He gave me a shot and asked me to wait for half an hour. I felt fine and he wrote a prescription on a sheet from his little pad. Luckily my husband was driving because I freaked out on the way home. My husband called the doctor and was told to take me to the hospital. That was the beginning of a two week stay in a locked drug ward. That is not the place to be for a fun vacation. I wasn't even allowed out of the area to go to the little shop on the first floor. My family and friends had to be let in through a locked door. My purse was searched. The only lethal weapon found was my fingernail file and it was removed.

My daughter's neighbor was head nurse in that department – not that it gave me any privileges – and she told me later the doctor ordered shots to 'quiet' me and I would put my head on the pillow and immediately pop up and say, "I've got to go to sleep"; then I would lay my head back on the pillow and suddenly I'd sit up to repeat, "I've got to go to sleep." That went on for two days. Those two days were washed completely out of my mind. I was "jailed" for two weeks. All I wanted was a good night's sleep and I didn't even get that! Needless to say that doctor-patient relationship ended.

I have suffered from loss of sleep all my life, going from one doctor to another, one treatment to another looking for the answer. I can understand the frustrations patients experience. My own life was described so aptly in a letter I received from a fellow sufferer that I can't state it more clearly:

I read an article in the Houston Chronicle *about "Restless Legs Syndrome (RLS) and I am more than grateful to find you-all. This is the first time I have ever heard that other people suffer with this malady. Not wishing this distress on anyone else. I sure am thankful to have someone to write or talk to about this. It's wonderful that now the ailment has a name. Everyone who has known me for any length of time truly believes I have lost my mind.*

I have arrived and departed in tears at the offices of family physicians, osteopaths, orthopedists, chiropractors, a neurosurgeon, masseuse, hypnotist, two acupuncture specialists, and even my ob-gyn. I have been x-rayed, MRIed, injected, rubbed and kneaded, hot packed, cold packed, pushed, pulled, shoved and twisted. At one point I was begging for surgery. Thank the Lord the neurosurgeon wouldn't do it. No one seems to have any knowledge and nothing has helped, at least not for very long.

My restlessness and pain are most severe at night. I would kill for six hours' straight sleep. Three or four hours is a treat. There are times the "feeling/pain/whatever" stays with me all day, from my hip to my ankle. I have been given drugs over the years with no long lasting relief. For the past year I am just living with it.

T. B., Houston, Texas

I sympathize with every patient who has been mistreated by misdiagnosis or given a doctor one-liner:

Never heard of it. You should exercise more.
It's only cramps in your legs. It will go away eventually.
We'll look into it.

                                                              E. P., Montreal, Quebec

The following sums up many of the letters:

Since everything is trial and error they should pay me to be a "guinea pig" I am at my "wits end." I told my doctor that there is a time bomb inside me that will blow up soon. . . . They don't want me to sleep during the day because that will mess up my sleeping during night. There have been many days which I go 22 hours without sleep. It has made me become "slap happy" and angry. When I tell the doctors, they honestly just look at me with a blank stare. I told one doctor yesterday that my life is just not worth living and I'm very, very scared to have this feeling. Virginia, I'm running on empty.

                                                              J. D., Glendale, California

One of my most frustrating experiences happened in 1981, five years before I had heard of RLS although I had been a victim of severe sleep deprivation for many years and physicians had tried every medication they could think of to help me sleep. I developed a kidney infection and I was swooped out of the doctor's office into the hospital before I knew what had happened. After undressing and getting into bed, I was given a shot immediately to get me settled. Settled? I hopped out of that bed and jumped up and down until a nurse forced me back into the bed and put the sides up. That did not deter me. I climbed over the sides. In came another nurse who gave me a second shot . . ."to quiet me." This went on and on until I was running up the halls with nurses telling me to get back to bed! I asked to be able to sit in a tub of warm water – over the years I had found this settled my nerves.

"It's too dangerous," a nurse replied.

"Not if you sit in the room with me." So began the night of shot and soak. I begged the nurses to stop the medication.

"Doctor's orders."

Since my doctor did not treat kidney problems he had called in a colleague, Dr. White, whom I had never met. Early the next morning the white-coated Dr. White, a most distinguished, handsome gentleman with white hair, swept into the room, shuffling papers and frowning like a king about to bestow his wisdom upon a serf. He said in a very serious voice, "I understand you were not very cooperative with the nurses last night."

"I told them not to give me a shot."

"But you needed help in calming yourself. You were very agitated and it certainly wasn't helping your kidney condition."

"I told them but they wouldn't listen. Said you had it on my the chart."

"M-m-m-m," he said shaking his head. "We have lots of testing to do today so do try to be cooperative." He turned to leave and I grabbed his coat sleeve and held on like a bulldog with a bone. He stopped. After all how many seventy-year old women clutch a sleeve and won't let go? He jerked his arm away and I held tighter.

"Now you listen to me, Doctor," I said. "You're just like all the rest around here. You don't want to listen to a darn thing a patient says. You've got rules, you've got your pills, your syringes, and you like to think you are very knowledgeable. You never asked why I walked and jumped around. I'll tell you why. I feel just like a little kid whose mother says, 'If you don't sit down I'll whack you,' and the kid says, 'Go ahead.' I can't sit still and I can't lie down. I feel like I am going to jump out of my skin. I want to scream and I would, except there are a lot of sick people here. Your medicine makes me want to explode! Do you understand? Explode!"

His pompous attitude changed. He drew up a chair. "Tell me about it," he said and listened. He sent for a neurologist. I had a brain scan. No problem (except fat fees for expert advice that wasn't very expert).

Together we began a year of searching for non-existent answers. But he listened and really tried. He retired and left me looking again for a kindly doctor who would listen. Four years later I found Dr. Herman Sessions. He prescribed medication for hyperactivity. He didn't know what was wrong with me, but he listened and he read medical journals. Finally he found the name of my disorder but could find no help.

My condition worsened. I became zombie-like, unable to do simple tasks. Without sleep my mind would shut down at inappropriate moments. We knew I had to get help. But where? There were few sleep disorders centers at that time. I told him of my son's suggestion that I go to a New York sleep center. He agreed. That began years of cooperation with my doctor for proper medication.

Today he sees many RLS patients, some of whom I have referred to him. Even though he is a general practitioner, actually a trained pediatrician, he understands that proper RLS care starts with and remains a close patient/doctor relationship. He has helped me through many bad times because beneath every physical problem I may have lies this hidden devil, the Sleep Thief, RLS. He can't cure it, but he surely does help make it tolerable.

The moral of this story is: Keep looking until you find a physician who will listen to your tale of woe. There **are** caring doctors, and there will be more when they learn about the seriousness of this disorder. They do exist. More and more I hear patients say things like this lady from Michigan: "I have a wonderful doctor now who takes plenty of time with anyone who sees him. He doesn't rush you in and out. I've gone to plenty of doctors so I know a good one from a bad one. I think he saved my life or at least my mind!"

It took over two years for me to be diagnosed. The VA thought I was a fraud. A neurologist knew immediately what it was. He had a 13-page research article that gave all of the details. The first paragraph was as though I had written it.

D. C., Spokane, Washington

We must not be too harsh in judging doctors who do not recognize RLS. Here is an example of one doctor's experience that she shared with us:

Restless Leg Syndrome Foundation: (September 26, 1994)

Thank you for your excellent efforts regarding Restless Leg Syndrome sufferers. I first was aware of the problem when a resident at the State Mental Hospital, when a young woman was admitted by her family because of her RLS problem. She developed helpless dependency on asylum life because of the severity of her RLS and resultant lack of ability to lead/form contacts for a normal social life. No one knew how to treat it; I tried all kinds of maneuvers to no avail. She didn't fit into any psychiatric category, but in those days we just sheltered her. Years later I read about RLS and looked her up to apologize for my lack of understanding. She was unsurprised – still dependent on being in a State Hospital system. She did not want to learn more.

Years after that I developed my own RLS, and my heart even more went out to her. My RLS is only positional-dependent on my earlier having spent at least an hour before retiring in a sitting position with my legs up (as propped up in bed, reading). I long to sit thus and read but I have learned I dare not because a sleepless night of walking ensues every time.

I wish you further good fortune in your work.

Virginia Truitt Sherr, M.D., F.A.P.A., Holland, Pennsylvania

We know there are many RLS patients out there being judged psychotics, hypochondriacs, malingers, and just plain crazy. All the years of being misdiagnosed and all the treatment programs we patients have endured should spark the RLS revolution. We should encourage medical schools to include RLS in the curricula. There is no excuse for this disorder being ignored in the classrooms. The word is out! RLS is a physical and treatable disorder. We must work together to ensure that the medical world is fully aware of this syndrome and its proper treatment so we can stop the Sleep Thief's ability to destroy our lives.

After my family physician exhausted medicine suggestions, he referred me to a neurologist, who sent me for an EEG. He said there were no abnormalities and he could find nothing wrong with me. For months thereafter, I was depressed and tried coping with the problem thinking I must be crazy. While going through some paper I happened upon a copy of the neurologist's original bill and saw his original diagnosis read "restless legs syndrome." That was the first clue I had and I relentlessly pursued it on my own thereafter.

C. B., Kingsport, Tennessee

There is information available for the RLS sufferer. The patient must learn the facts about the disorder that is destroying his or her life! It is most important to arm oneself with the armor of knowledge before going on the hunt for a doctor who can help. It is vital that physicians be made aware of their ignorance of this disorder. RLS vigilantes must broadcast the message. Taking a cue from the successful "Learn to Read Program," each one must teach one or two or three, even if one of the number is a physician. Gone must be the days of being laughed at. This malady is not a laughing matter even if the name brings forth a snicker or two from friend or foe.

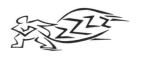

Breaking the "Patient" Mode

Carol Upchurch Walker
Member of the Board of Directors of the RLS Foundation

I have what is considered to be a very severe case of RLS, but for six years I was told, and I believed, that I had Multiple Sclerosis (MS). I did not come by this diagnosis easily. I had searched for 20 years for an answer to my medical problems. I saw doctors from Maine to California, and from Key West, Florida, to Newport, Rhode Island, and no one was sure what plagued me. I settled in the Northeast in the mid 1980s. With the approval and referral of my family physician, I decided to seek help from the top specialist in every field that seemed relevant to my continuing problems. Five specialists agreed that I suffered from MS. I was relieved to finally have a diagnosis even though I was not happy to "have" what they found. But at least I could stop looking: I could begin treatment, and possibly get better.

This is not what happened, however. I did begin to be cared for by a top MS specialist. I received medication that was supposed to relieve my symptoms. I sought out patient support groups, for my mental health and better understanding. I studied and read everything I could find about this disease, MS, so I could be an informed patient and keep my family, loved ones, and friends up to date on my condition and prognosis.

Time passed and I became very disillusioned, as the treatments and medication did not help me at all. Many obvious symptoms, (restlessness and inability to sleep) from which I continued to suffer, were being ignored as if they did not exist. The support groups were no help because I did not "connect" with the other MS patients in any way. Their problems and complaints seemed foreign to me, as mine did to them. We had nothing in common. Whenever I questioned these things, nothing was looked into or rechecked. I was simply told that I was "in denial."

I found a magazine article concerning a neurological disorder that my symptoms fit the descriptions perfectly. I took it to my neurologist and I was told that it was merely a coincidence. I began to ask about RLS and I later found out that neither the doctor nor any of my other doctors knew anything about RLS.

In early 1991, after experiencing extreme physical problems for a few days, my group of specialists decided to hospitalize me. The admittance sheet stated the reason for hospitalization as "exacerbation of MS." I spent five days as an inpatient. Each of the specialists, whose care I was under, visited me, ordered tests, and wrote up progress reports; but not one of them actually listened to my explanation of the symptoms I was feeling. Each night I was given a sleeping pill – but rather than producing sleep, the pills had the opposite effect, and I felt electrified. My restless legs drove me wild, and I was unable to remain in bed. The halls circled around the nurses' station. For five nights, from 11 p.m. to 5 o'clock the next morning, I walked those halls, around and around and around. At first the nurses questioned why I wasn't in bed. I'm sure they assumed I was crazy, then they simply ignored me. That I did not sleep even one hour out of the five nights I was hospitalized never made it into my record; that fact was absolutely ignored. When I related this to doctors each morning, seeing no notes from the nurses concerning this matter, I think they thought I was imagining my need to walk. When I checked out of the hospital the dismissal sheet stated, "MS now under control." It was at this time that I knew for sure that, after six years of being treated for it, I did not have and had never had Multiple Sclerosis.

I felt anger, frustration, disbelief, distrust, and a lot of other emotions; but at the same time, I felt relief. I became more determined than ever to find out what disease I was suffering from. I wondered if I could ever trust a doctor again. What I did decide to do was to trust my own instincts about my health and my body, and to have belief in myself and my own intuition.

Sleep Disorder Centers began to open throughout the nation. More and more information began to circulate about the good they were doing. So I took a risk, answered an advertisement in the newspaper for sleep study patients and a very prestigious clinic accepted me. After one perfectly miserable night in the sleep lab I was diagnosed as having the *Restless Legs Syndrome* – an answer I had been seeking for 26 years. I was convinced that this was a true and correct diagnosis. Finally knowing "what I had" was like seeing a light at the end of a long, dark tunnel. I felt ecstatic! But how could I contend with my mistrust of doctors and my anger for lost years?

After a lot of soul searching, I slowly realized that no doctor intentionally misdiagnoses a patient. It would certainly not be in his/her best interests to do so. And from my experience with misdiagnosis, I understood that a doctor who finally makes a correct diagnosis of a disease never blames his/her colleagues, because someday or time he/she might misjudge an unknown and baffling medical problem.

A doctor is always "practicing" and can only put his best knowledge to use by listening to the patients' symptoms and complaints. The results of medical tests are only as useful as the available information at the time and place. In my case, the correct medical information for a correct diagnosis was not widely available. Even though for a six year period I was wrongly tested by the medical profession, no harm was ever intended for me and, except for my own misery, none was ever done to me.

So I chose to simply tell each of the fine doctors who diagnosed me incorrectly that I had been re-diagnosed with RLS. They were very gracious. I thanked each one of them for their interest and care and I moved on. I was not disappointed. All of the doctors told me how very sorry they were that they had not known more at the time. They wished me well and offered to help me in any way they could in the future, if necessary. I also wished them well. I am learning anew to trust doctors and to realize that they can only do the best they know how at the time, and that I, not the doctor, am completely responsible for my own health and well-being.

For so long, the people who suffered with the symptoms of this disorder thought they were all alone. That is why the information contained in this book is so important to both the medical community and to the lay person who needs to know more about the condition known as *Restless Legs Syndrome.* This subject has not been taught in medical schools. I have a 93-year-old uncle, who is a medical doctor and a sufferer of RLS. He had never heard of any treatment for this disease during his medical career. He was unable to find help for himself or for his mother, my grandmother, also an RLS victim.

I have learned a great deal from being misdiagnosed. Today, I behave differently with a doctor. I tend not to be quite as "patient." I am clearly more assertive and insist on more control of my own care. I take more responsibility for myself and my disease. I make an attempt to know as much, or more, as the doctor treating me. I know that I must remain a diligent investigator and continue to learn everything possible in order to assist the medical profession in my case. I consider myself and my doctor to be a team. If I do not take these important steps in working with the professional medical personnel, then I am as culpable as the doctor if I receive less than excellent treatment.

Chapter Two

The Search for Treatment of RLS

by Wayne A. Hening, M.D., Ph.D.

History of Treatment of RLS and Overview of RLS Therapy

First writing in Latin in 1672 (with later translation into English for a book published in 1685,) Sir Thomas Willis, a noted British biologist and physician, described a patient who had difficulty sleeping because of discomfort in the limbs. He noted that she was calm in the daytime, but bothered by her symptoms whenever she took to bed and tried to rest. Sleep was impossible, since her limbs leaped about and she experienced "unquietness" and "cramps," which could be aptly described as "torture." Willis likened her to someone on the "Rack." Fortunately, her "convulsive distempers" were relieved by a large dose of laudanum, an extract of the opium poppy that was one of the ancestors of the present day opiate-like medications. Many of us have noted that her condition sounds like a severe case of RLS and even today, we use opiate-like medications (see Section II, chapter 3, Medications Helpful in RLS) to relieve RLS. Willis, for whom the important ring of major arteries at the base of the brain, the Circle of Willis, is named, was also a lucky physician, for after several months of treatment, his case of the RLS remitted and he could claim a "cure," an outcome which usually eludes us today. Most of us, both treating physicians and patients, find that RLS is an intermittent or chronic condition and that treatment will be required over many years.

After Willis, there were a few scattered reports of conditions resembling RLS in the literature, but it was almost three centuries later that Karl Ekbom, a Swedish physician, wrote a long monograph on RLS. Ekbom's work began the modern era in the understanding and treatment of RLS. For his pivotal work, the condition is at times named after him as Ekbom's syndrome.

Ekbom believed that RLS was caused by poor circulation in the legs. Therefore, he recommended medications that might increase the blood flow by expanding the arteries (vasodilators). In his hands, these medications were said to be quite helpful. In later years, they have fallen into disuse and no formal studies were ever done to prove their effectiveness. Today, most experts do not think that RLS is primarily caused by poor circulation, but cold feet are common in RLS patients and abnormal blood flow may be a part of the overall picture of RLS. More recently, Dr. Sonia Ancoli-Israel found that some patients are relieved by behavioral techniques that increase blood flow in the legs.

Ekbom also recognized that opiate-like medications or sedatives, such as barbiturates, could help patients with RLS. However, he felt that these medications caused too many problems, such as addiction, that made their use more harmful than helpful. In the decades which followed Ekbom's first publication, there were an increasing number of reports dealing with the clinical picture, cause, and treatment of RLS. A number of different types of medications that act on the central nervous system were first suggested as useful for RLS, including propranolol (Inderal), a beta-blocker which counteracts the effects of adrenalin and noradrenalin, and is generally used to treat high blood pressure, tremor, and stage fright! Diazepam (Valium), a member of the benzodiazepine family of sedatives, was also recommended. Because RLS was found to be more common in those with low blood count (anemia), iron to build up the blood was also recommended as were various vitamin treatments, such as folic acid or vitamin E.

Since the late 1970s there has been a growing interest in the study of RLS and its treatment. One important discovery that helped pave the way to this increased interest was the recognition by Dr. Elio Lugaresi and his colleagues in the 1960s that many people with RLS also have Periodic Limb Movements in Sleep (PLMS). These are regularly recurring movements, usually in the legs, that can wake RLS patients when they fall asleep. In general, it has been found that medications which relieve RLS also reduce PLMS. Because periodic limb movements (PLMs) are easy to recognize and count, medical investigators began to use them to gauge whether a medication was helpful for RLS patients and those with PLMS alone (a condition known as Periodic Limb Movement Disorder, PLMD).

A new era in RLS therapy has been ushered in since 1980 through the use of controlled studies in which medications felt to be helpful for RLS are tested against placebo medication. To make sure that no subtle suggestions influence the outcome of these studies, they are done in a double blind fashion. Neither the people running the study (one blind) nor the patient (second blind) knows whether the pills the patient is taking are the drug itself or a placebo. Only the pharmacist who is making up the pills knows whether the patient is receiving the experimental medication or the placebo. Based on this type of sophisticated clinical trial, a number of the medications that I will discuss in the next chapter have been shown to be helpful for at least some aspects of RLS and PLMS. These medications include benzodiazepines; dopaminergic agents – drugs active on the dopamine system of the brain; opiate-like medications; cabamazepine (Tegretol), a medication for epilepsy; baclofen (Lioresal), a muscle relaxant; and clonidine (Catapres), a medication also used for high blood pressure. Other medications have been studied in less formal ways and new medications are just being discovered. Gabapentin (Neurontin), a drug used primarily to control seizures, was recently reported to be helpful for RLS. I will discuss all these medications in greater detail in the following chapter.

There are, therefore, a fair number of medications today that may be useful for RLS. In the future, this number may well grow and as we know more about medications, their usefulness and limitations, we will be better able to decide which are the best medications for RLS. Of course, in the future, our whole idea of treating RLS may change. If a gene for RLS is discovered, many new vistas for therapy may open up, including the eventual possibility of a "genetic" cure. Until that happens, however, the best chance for the RLS patient to get safe and proper relief is to wisely use the medications available today, after deciding if they are needed. The rest of this chapter will discuss how the patient can work with a knowledgeable or "educable" physician to secure a personally satisfying therapeutic outcome.

In the next chapter, I will introduce the different types of medications in use today, their strong points and their drawbacks. Finally, in the following chapter, I will suggest some current schemes for how to manage treatment of RLS derived from my personal experience and that of my colleague, Dr. Arthur S. Walters, the work of the group at Johns Hopkins, including Drs. Richard Allen, David Buchholz, and Christopher Earley; and the results of a survey on RLS therapy nationwide and internationally that was conducted by our group at the Lyons VA Medical Center under the auspices of the Clemente Foundation.

Dr. Daniel Picchietti has taken a particular interest in studying RLS when it appears in children and how it should be approached in that age group. Since his chapter in this book (Section I, Chapter 8) thoroughly covers treatment of children with RLS, I will not duplicate that subject here. All those interested in the problem of treating childhood RLS should turn to his chapter.

At the outset, I must state that I have my own biases. I treat patients whose RLS is sufficiently severe that it is not manageable with everyday, non-pharmacological maneuvers. I have also seen that medications can work quite well and over periods of many years (ten or more) provide a far more comfortable life for patients with RLS, without apparent serious side effects. But I recognize that for many people, taking medications for RLS may not be necessary. Many patients can make their symptoms tolerable by the correct amount of sleep and exercise, avoiding caffeine, or simple maneuvers such as a brief turn on the exercise bicycle or a hot shower before bedtime. Other patients report to me a wide variety of dietary, holistic, or other practices that they believe provide them with adequate relief. I encourage any such tricks and experiments and encourage patients to avoid medication if they can, but not to become martyrs to their illness when medication can provide relief. Finally, my experience with medications, both in my own practice and in the literature, although considerable, is not unlimited. I have had more experience with some medications than others. Compared to someone else, I may have had more or less success with a particular medication. Therefore, I may emphasize some medications more than is their due and slight others. Please take what I say then with a grain of salt for what I am presenting to you is one man's knowledge and experience, not the ultimate word on how you should treat your RLS symptoms.

Some General Guidelines in Obtaining Treatment for RLS

In what follows, I discuss more or less how I would want my own good friend or relative to approach the treatment of a chronic disorder such as RLS. From that point of view, it is not dissimilar to the approach needed for the treatment of any other significant disorder that is likely to persist, such as chronic lung disease or multiple sclerosis – to name just two examples. It also emphasizes some of my treatment biases, which I will explain in a later chapter but which are also to a large degree common to many experts now treating RLS.

The first key to successful treatment is to find a physician whom you trust and with whom you can work. You should feel free to speak with the physician and to ask questions. The physician should take enough time to get to know you, to understand how RLS affects you, and to understand what matters to you in obtaining treatment. This is necessary if you are to receive individualized treatment that is tailored to your own lifestyle and preferences.

It is also important that the physician either understand RLS or be willing to learn about the condition. More and more physicians, particularly those with an interest in sleep, do have some expertise in treating RLS, but it is clear that not just any physician is likely to be familiar with the condition and its treatment. Finding someone with expertise may take a bit of work. You might discuss treatment with people at a local RLS support group or ask the RLS Foundation for a list of sleep centers or other doctors more likely to be knowledgeable about RLS. If your referral is only to a neurologist or sleep center, try to find out from the office staff or the doctor whether he or she is familiar with RLS, before going for an appointment.

In many cases, you may not be able to find any doctor near your home who can help you who already is an expert in RLS. This would probably be true today for the majority of people in the country. In that case, you may find a doctor who is willing to learn about RLS who might read the publications of the RLS Foundation, professional papers on RLS, or a chapter such as this. Perhaps you might go some distance for an initial consultation and report, which could then be sent back to a local doctor, whether internist, family physician, or neurologist, who will carry out the day-to-day adjustment of medications. In the near future, such options as Tel-med, the ability to obtain electronic consultations from a remote site, may allow primary care physicians to obtain on-line advice from experts. Other modes of rapid provision of information may also make information about RLS, like that about other conditions, much more easily available to primary care physicians.

Third, I think it is important to develop a working partnership with the doctor who is going to take care of your RLS. Some cases of RLS are simple, and not especially severe, and may stay that way. An occasional medication to relieve a bad day or a difficult outing may be the most that is needed. However, other cases of RLS can be very severe and substantially impair the quality of the patient's life. The more severe your condition, the more important it is to work with the doctor to obtain the best relief possible for you. In such cases, it may be necessary to try several medications or a combination of different medications in order to obtain optimal relief. In addition, medications that work for a while may cease to work effectively. In that case, new medications may need to be tried or a new medication added to your current regimen. Finally, as we learn more about RLS there may be new therapies that can be considered as a substitute or in addition to a regimen that is working. Or we may find that, in the long run, some therapies we now endorse have unanticipated drawbacks. For better or worse, this is a pioneering era for the treatment of RLS and the current generation of patients may see more changes in what is the "conventional wisdom" regarding the treatment of RLS than any previous generation or any generation to come.

Once you have found a knowledgeable physician with whom you can work, the next question is How to treat your RLS? The very first question of treatment is whether any medication is needed at all. Many patients can manage with proper exercise, diet, and sleep hygiene to sufficiently limit their RLS symptoms so that no medication is needed. Or the symptoms may be so mild that no assistance is necessary. But it may be that your symptoms are so severe that they do impair your quality of life and nothing you can do seems to keep them sufficiently under control. Then you will probably want to obtain medication, but maybe you won't need medication every day. Perhaps you are only bothered by long dinner parties or plane or bus trips or an occasional day when the legs just won't stop. Then you may only need a "prn" medication, one that can be used only when needed. Many of the medications used for RLS can be used on a "prn" basis, but some important ones, such as pergolide (Permax), cannot be so used.

If your RLS occurs most days (or nights!), then you probably will need a medication that is taken on a daily basis. Choosing a medication may then require balancing between the benefits that the medication can provide and the side-effects or other drawbacks of treatment. In general, I recommend beginning most medications at a low dose and then building them up gradually until adequate benefit is obtained, side effects emerge, or a maximum reasonable dose is reached. Starting slow and building up slowly often limits the side effects. In addition, since the effects of long term use of most medications prescribed for RLS is largely unknown, it is prudent to select the lowest effective dose for treatment. This may be most easily determined if the dose is built up gradually. Each medication has a generally recommended or suggested range. However, in selected cases, if the medication is otherwise working, higher than recommended doses can be used. This must be decided between physician and patient, but in some cases, patients clearly have benefited from doses higher than those customarily employed.

I should add one other concern. Some restless legs patients will have other medical or psychiatric disorders or be taking additional medications. The doctor who treats the RLS must take these into account, because some RLS medicines may not be compatible with other disorders or medications. For example, propranolol (Inderal) needs to be used very cautiously in patients with lung disease or diabetes and may cause excessively low blood pressure, hypotension, in patients taking other medicines for high blood pressure. On the other hand, an RLS medication may also sometimes be beneficial for another condition. For example, clonidine (Catapres) or propranolol (Inderal) can benefit both RLS and high blood pressure. It may be possible to coordinate your care so that one medicine adequately treats both your medical problem and your RLS. To make sure possible drug interactions are considered, I believe it is always a good idea to take your medications or a list of them with you when you go for a consultation. The consulting doctor can then review them before prescribing additional therapy. You should also know or have records that indicate the important features of your medical history.

What do you do when a medication does not work or has too troubling a set of side effects? If the medication is minimally effective or ineffective or if side effects are intolerable, then it is probably necessary to switch to another medication. As discussed in the next chapter, several different types of medications may help in RLS. If you haven't responded well to one type of medication, you might try another type. Sometimes, even medications of the same type may have very different properties. For example, two medications that work on the dopamine system, the combination of L-DOPA and carbidopa (Sinemet) and pergolide (Permax) have somewhat different side effects. If a medication is working to some degree and can be tolerated at some doses, but does not provide full relief, then different solutions might be considered. It may still be best to switch to a completely different medication. In general, if all the problems can be solved with a single medication, that is the simplest and probably the optimal solution. In some cases, the strengths add together but the side effects do not. So combination therapy is something to be at least considered when no single medication gives adequate relief. Usually, combination therapy involves choosing medications of different types – a benzodiazepine along with an opioid, for example. I have found that severe RLS may require medications of three different types.

One special kind of treatment is "symptomatic" therapy. This is used for cases where RLS is caused by another medical abnormality. One common abnormality that may cause RLS is anemia, "thin blood" due to an insufficient quantity of red blood cells. The most common type of anemia associated with RLS is due to inadequate iron in the blood. Iron is needed for the oxygen carrying pigment, hemoglobin. If iron is deficient, it can lead to an underproduction of the red blood cells needed to carry oxygen bound to hemoglobin. This, in turn, leads to anemia, which can be detected by the doctor in a complete blood count. Further tests can determine that the amount of iron and of its carrying protein, ferritin, is inadequate. Replacing iron may then relieve the anemia and "cure" the "symptomatic" RLS. Vitamins for RLS may play a similar role, although clear cut deficits are less likely to be shown. Another kind of therapy in RLS is "avoidance" therapy. Some medications may increase RLS symptoms, rather than relieve them. This may be true of a number of antidepressant medications as well as some of the major tranquilizers used to treat psychiatric illness. Other medications may temporarily relieve RLS symptoms, but cause the symptoms to increase later on as levels of the medication drop. Dr. Richard Allen of Johns Hopkins has told me that this may be true of caffeine, which may provide temporary relief of RLS soon after it is consumed, but then cause symptoms to return later, perhaps more strongly, as its effects wear off.

Finally, I want to just briefly touch on a few issues of therapy that need to be considered for an RLS patient: when to take medications, whether to rotate medications, and how to stop medications. Usually, medications should be taken to anticipate symptoms. For example, if your leg problems begin as soon as you go to bed, the time to take the medication is somewhat less than a half hour for many medications but longer for some (an hour or more for extended release form of combined L-DOPA and carbidopa [Sinemet CR]). If the legs go crazy after dinner, then something taken with or even before the meal might be appropriate. Sometimes medications will last a certain period of time and then wear off. This often occurs when L-DOPA and carbidopa combination (Sinemet) is taken at bedtime. If you then wake several hours later with the legs going again, another dose of medication could well be appropriate. If your symptoms are bad, they may bother you throughout most of the day.

In that case, you may need to take medications at intervals all day long. The time between doses should be adjusted so that the leg symptoms are kept quiet. This may require a different adjustment for each medication and each patient. And even when a patient is taking a regular medication, there may be times when an extra dose is needed, such as before a long trip.

These are all issues of timing that are best worked out in a collaborative effort with the treating physician. Another option that is sometimes considered is rotating medications: spending two or three weeks taking one type of medication, then switching to another. The rationale for this approach is that medications sometimes lose efficacy with time. It seems as if the body adjusts to them and not only are side effects diminished, but the very therapeutic results for which they are taken. Personally, I have not found that diminishing benefit is such a problem that rotation is often necessary, so I have little experience with it. But it is something to think about if a patient responds well to several medications, but then shortly loses the benefit. **Finally, it is important to remember that for some medications, it is important that they not be stopped abruptly.** This is particularly true if medications have been taken for a period of time, with frequent doses, and at a high dose level. Combined L-DOPA and carbidopa (Sinemet) as well as other dopaminergic medications and beta-blockers such as propranolol (Inderal) may cause significant medical complications if they are stopped abruptly, as may high dose benzodiazepines or high dose opioids. When in doubt, medications should be tapered over a period of a week or more so that the body adjusts gradually to their withdrawal.

Wayne A. Hening, M.D., Ph.D.
Department of Neurology
Robert Wood Johnson Medical School
University of Medicine and Dentistry of New Jersey
New Brunswick, New Jersey

Chapter Three

Medications Helpful in RLS

Wayne A. Hening, M.D., Ph.D.

For simplicity, I have broken down the medications currently used in RLS into four classes: primary medications, those most likely to help the RLS patient; secondary medications, those which may be worth a try, but which have not been shown to be as successful or studied as carefully as the medications in the primary class; symptomatic medications, those aimed at particular causes for RLS; and finally, medications to avoid. I also add a few words on non-pharmacological therapy.

I want again to stress that my review is colored by my particular biases and that I know, from the Clemente study[1] that some physicians who treat many RLS patients would take a quite different point of view. In addition, what I write today is valid for 1996, and, in part, for the years after, but five or ten years from now, what I have to say in this section of the chapter is likely to be obsolete and may even be completely wrong. So if you are reading this chapter in

---

[1] Clemente Foundation RLS Therapy Study in Section II, Chapter 4.

the year 2003, check a more recent reference before deciding that a medication I mention is just what you want to have prescribed.

I also want to stress that what is presented here is a sketch. It is necessarily incomplete. Treatment should always be undertaken together with a doctor who can assess your general health, your particular reaction to medications, your other medical problems and medications, to be sure that a particular medication poses no particular risk in your individual case.

To avoid confusion on medication names, I will use generic and brand names for all medications when I first mention a medication in a given part of the chapter. The generic name is that typically used in medical writing. It is not as elaborate as the full chemical name, but there is only a single generic name for a chemical compound used as a medication. There may be many different brand names for the same compound. For example, Motrin, Nuprin, and Advil are all brand names for the compound whose generic name is ibuprofen. In this chapter and the later one on treatment strategies, I have linked the generic name to the most common brand names, since people often hear first or only recognize the common brand names. For example, most people know the brand Sinemet of combined L-DOPA with carbidopa. I will also try to clarify the different forms of a common medication, such as L-DOPA since the same active ingredient may be packaged or combined in different ways.

I also give dose ranges of medications as a rough guide in the kinds of doses that are taken. These are not rigid limits: some doctors may prescribe smaller or larger doses and are perfectly correct. Also, please note that the dose of one medication cannot be compared to that of another medication. Some medications are stronger, even if of the same type. For example, a common dose of the benzodiazepine, triazolam (Halcion) is one quarter of a milligram (0.25 mg). Another benzodiazepam medication, temazepam (Restoril) is typically taken in a thirty milligram (30 mg) dose. The temazepam is not 120 times stronger, but is only about an equivalent dose. It takes a much larger quantity of the temazepam to be as strong as the triazolam. To save space, I will use the abbreviation "mg" for milligrams. Note that a milligram is one thousandth of a gram. A gram is roughly one twenty-eighth part of an ounce. Some medications, such as pergolide (Permax) are usually taken in fractions of a milligram.

Primary treatment

The types of medications included within primary treatment have two important features. First, their ability to help all or most of the problems of RLS patients has been established in well controlled double blind studies. Therefore, we know that they can work. Second, there has been a fair amount of experience in the use of these medications to treat RLS, so that many sleep doctors are familiar with using them. The general feeling is that these medications are helpful and can be used with relative safety. This does not mean, however, that every medicine of each type is equally effective or has been as thoroughly tested. Nor does it mean that each of these medications will work for the RLS patient. I will discuss in turn primary medications of the sedative type like clonazepam (Klonopin), which are in the benzodiazepine class; medications that act upon the nervous system neuro-transmitter-chemical, dopamine, which can be called dopaminergic medications, including combined L-DOPA with carbidopa (Sinemet); and opiate-like medications, generally known as opioids, which are pain-killing medications of the narcotic type.

Benzodiazepines:

Sedating medications are useful for treatment of both RLS and PLMS. Ekbom in 1945 recognized the usefulness of sedatives in treating RLS, especially barbiturates such as phenobarbital. Strang first reported the use of a benzodiazepine, diazepam (Valium) for RLS in the 1960s. The basic advantage of the benzodiazepines over other sedatives is that they are safer. Taken alone, the benzodiazepines can cause drowsiness or even stupor and coma if taken in excess, but even doses far above the therapeutic range are unlikely to be lethal. However, combined with other sedatives, including alcohol, they can be much more dangerous. The strong point of the benzodiazepines in the treatment of RLS is in improving the quality of sleep. They may also benefit waking symptoms in RLS, but this is less well-established. They seem to decrease the number of PLMS, but not as much as the other two primary types of medication. The most used benzodiazepine is clonazepam (Klonopin), usually taken at or near bed time. One advantage of clonazepam is that it is helpful for other motor disorders of sleep, which may be common in older patients. For instance, it appears to be quite beneficial for a particular malady of the dreaming stage of sleep, Rapid Eye Movement (REM) Sleep Behavior Disorder. In this condition patients appear to be acting out their dreams and may end up striking their bed partners or even injuring themselves by jumping out of bed. Typical doses of some of the benzodiazepines have been: clonazepam (Klonopin) in doses of 0.5 to 2 mg; temazepam (Restoril) in doses of 15 to 45 mg; and triazolam (Halcion) in doses of 0.125 to 0. 5 mg. All are usually taken before bedtime. The doses may also be divided, with some reserved for later in the night. Doses for daytime treatment of RLS are less well established. Diazepam (Valium) has also been for daytime symptoms; a typical dose might be 5 mg twice a day. Drawbacks include the potential for confusion or daytime sleepiness, especially in older patients. As benzodiazepines are taken over a number of days, some of them – such as diazepam or clonazepam – can accumulate, especially in older patients and cause confusion or other mental changes. This must be carefully monitored, although at the doses mentioned in this paragraph, it has not usually been a significant problem.

Dopaminergic Agents:

These medications all act upon the dopamine system of the central nervous system. Dopaminergic refers to those nerve cells which use dopamine. The central nervous system consists of the brain within the skull and the spinal cord within the spine. Dopamine is one of the chemicals called "neurotransmitters" that nerve cells use to communicate with each other. The typical nerve cell has a round, oval, or pyramid-shaped cell body from which a variety of projections emerge. The cell's axon is the projection which carries the cell's message to other cells. Shaped like a cable, but often branching, especially near its end, the axon can project from one cell only to nearby cells or to entirely different parts of the brain or spinal cord. Some axons even travel the length of the spinal cord, between the base of the spine and the brain. It is now known that there are several important pathways in the central nervous system in which dopamine containing cells send axons from one part to another. One of these pathways, the nigrostriatal, withers away in Parkinson's disease. Two other pathways, the mesolimbic and mesofrontal, may be disordered in schizophrenia. There is also a dopamine pathway that descends from the bottom part of the brain, the brainstem, down into the spinal cord; that pathway may help stimulate walking. It is strongly suspected by many researchers that the dopamine system is important for the symptoms of RLS. It is not known, however, which pathways are involved in RLS nor how the involved pathways affect RLS symptoms. To see whether dopamine pathways might be abnormal in the brains of RLS patients, Dr. Walters of the RLS Medical Advisory Board and Dr. David Eidelberg of Northshore Hospital in New York conducted a preliminary brain imaging study of RLS patients using PET (Positron Emission Tomography). They injected a radioactive substance, fluorodopa, that is taken up from the blood by dopamine nerve cells. Using the PET machine, they then developed a brain image or picture of the brain which showed how active the nerve cells were in taking up the fluorodopa. No abnormal nerve cell activity was found in the RLS patients. However, the abnormality in RLS may be subtle or located in the lower regions of the central nervous system, the brainstem and spinal cord, which could not be imaged in that PET study.

Dopamine-related medications are useful for treatment of both RLS and PLMS. They improve all features of RLS including subjective discomfort, dyskinesias while awake, PLMS, and sleep quality. There are two main types of dopamine-related medications. Dopamine precursors are medications that the central nervous system can convert into the active compound, dopamine. Dopamine agonists act directly, they take the place of dopamine and stimulate the same cells that dopamine would stimulate. They make these cells believe they are receiving a message from the dopamine nerve cells. Dopamine precursors have been used most extensively for the treatment of RLS. In the United States, they come as a combination of L-DOPA, the precursor itself, and carbidopa, a related compound which blocks the premature conversion of L-DOPA to dopamine before it enters the central nervous system. This is important for two reasons. First, if the L-DOPA is converted to dopamine before it enters the central nervous system, less of it will be available to be used by nerve cells. Second, the dopamine circulating in the blood may cause unpleasant side effects, such as nausea or vomiting, that dopamine in the nervous system would not cause. The combination of the L-DOPA with carbidopa is available either as a regular release (Sinemet) or sustained release compound (Sinemet CR). (Outside the United States, the compound may include benserazide, instead of carbidopa. The combination of L-DOPA with benserazide has a brand name Madopar.) The sustained release form of the compound (Sinemet CR) is more slowly taken up into the body and lasts longer. Both regular and slow release compounds indicate how much L-DOPA and carbidopa is in each pill. They have two numbers separated by a slash, such as 10/100 or 50/200. The first number always indicates the milligrams of carbidopa in the pill and the second number, the milligrams of L-DOPA. Your pharmacy may list the medication as carbidopa/levodopa. Levodopa is just another variant of the name L-DOPA. Typical doses of the regular release compound are from 10/100, 25/100 to 100/400 (as an example 25/100 means 25 milligrams of carbidopa with 100 milligrams of L-DOPA). The patient takes these pills in divided doses before bedtime or before bedtime and during the night. Because it takes approximately 75 milligrams of carbidopa for an effective block of L-DOPA conversion, patients on the low dose combination may not get enough carbidopa. This problem can be alleviated by using combinations with relatively more carbidopa (Sinemet 25/100 instead of 10/100). Additional pure carbidopa can also be given.

Two main problems have been noted with the use of these combination medications: "rebound," the tendency of symptoms to recur late in the night or in the early morning leading to poor sleep quality near morning and "augmentation," the tendency for symptoms to develop earlier in the day (e.g., morning or late afternoon instead of mid-evening) and to be more severe than before treatment. Side effects include gastrointestinal discomfort, nausea and vomiting, or headache. Confusion and other mental changes occur fairly commonly in patients with Parkinson's disease taking these medications, but seems to be quite rare in RLS.

Sustained release preparations last longer, but may take longer to become active (up to one and a half hours compared to one half hour for the regular preparation). Therefore, sustained release should be taken earlier than the regular release to be fully active by bedtime. In some patients, because symptoms occur throughout the day or develop throughout the day after treatment, L-DOPA with carbidopa may be taken regularly both day and night. This dosing schedule may be effective, but unless the patient already had such wide-spread symptoms before therapy, the need for around-the-clock dosages probably indicates that a different medication should be tried. Both regular and sustained release L-DOPA with carbidopa can be taken on a "prn" basis, just when needed. This is one advantage that the compound has over the dopamine agonist, pergolide (Permax), which seems to offer a good alternative but cannot be taken effectively on a "prn" basis.

The combination of L-DOPA with carbidopa is usually taken by patients with Parkinson's disease, many of whom use higher doses than those common for treatment of RLS. After a number of years of such treatment, patient response may diminish and abnormal involuntary movements, dyskinesias, can occur and sometimes be quite severe. These can be evanescent, jumpy movements (choreiform movements), or slower, twisting or sustained movements (dystonic movements). Long-term treatment has not led often to these kinds of abnormal movements in patients with RLS treated with the combination. It is currently believed that such complications are unlikely, since the dopamine system in RLS is probably not depleted in the way that it is in Parkinson's disease. However, this possible risk should be acknowledged and doses of the combination, as well as other dopamine related agents, should be kept as low as feasible.

Two dopamine agonists, bromocriptine (Paralodel) and pergolide (Permax), have been tried successfully in RLS and PLMS. Typical doses for therapy have been 5 to 15 mg of bromocriptine or 0.10 to 0.6 mg of pergolide, either drug taken in divided doses before bedtime. In some patients, considerably higher doses of all these drugs have been tried when lower doses did not work. The agonists do not seem to show to the same degree the problems of rebound and augmentation seen with L-DOPA based combinations. Nasal stuffiness (especially with pergolide), gastrointestinal discomfort, and low blood pressure (which can cause fainting) have occurred as side effects. Particularly with pergolide, the dose must be carefully increased (beginning with only 0.05 mg per day and then increasing every several days until an effective dose is reached) to avoid low blood pressure or other side effects. Our group (led by Dr. Arthur Walters, Chairman of the Medical Advisory Board) reported excellent results with bromocriptine in a controlled study. Other groups have tried it informally and some have not been impressed at its efficacy. Pergolide has also been tried recently by a number of groups. There are no formal publications of controlled studies establishing its efficacy, but all indicated that it was quite beneficial.

Opioids:

Opioids are synthetic compounds which act like the natural opiates. Natural opiates include codeine and morphine, chemicals derived from the poppy plant. These chemicals all induce sedation or sleep and, therefore, are called narcotics (meaning sleep-inducing compounds). As mentioned earlier, in the seventeenth century Willis successfully used an opiate-like medication, laudanum, to treat a condition that sounds like RLS.

Ekbom was aware of their efficacy, but felt that their chronic use was problematic. The brain has its own natural opiate-like substances, called endogenous opiates, which are found in brain cells and act as neurotransmitters. Because experiments have shown that agents which block opioid action prevent these medications from helping RLS, it is believed that opioid medications work via the endogenous opiate system. It is also known that the endogenous opiate system acts upon the dopamine system in the brain. Some experiments have suggested that the opioid medications may act through the dopamine system. These narcotic medications are clearly useful for treating RLS and probably are also effective for PLMS. Many different opioids have been tried informally, including codeine, propoxyphene (Darvon), oxycodone (in Percodan), pentazocine (Talwin), and methadone (roughly graded from mild to strong). Doses have been quite variable, but typical doses used for patients have been: codeine, 15 to 240 mg per day; propoxyphene (Darvon), 130 to 520 mg per day; oxycodone (Percodan or Percocet), 2.5 to 20 mg per day; pentazocine (Talwin), 50 to 200 mg per day; and methadone, 5 to 30 mg per day. Opioids are taken at the times when symptoms are expected, either in the evening and at night or throughout the day. Methadone, which has such a long half-life, can usually be taken once a day. Opioids can also be taken on a "prn" basis, such as before going to a movie theater or a support group meeting. In the future, additional opioids may be used. Some others have long half lives, as does methadone, or can be used as a patch with gradual release.

Our group at the Lyons VA Medical Center and the UMDNJ-Robert Wood Johnson Medical School found clinical benefit to subjective symptoms, sleep measures, and PLMS with oxycodone at a mean dose of 15.9 mg per day, whereas the Johns Hopkins group in a double blind study of propoxyphene napsylate (Darvon-N), 300 mg per night found benefits to subjective symptoms and total motor activity, but no statistically significant reduction in PLMs. One study of patients with PLMS alone found that some responded to opioids.

The major worry with the use of narcotic medication is addiction. This worry is probably almost always exaggerated for RLS patients. As with other patients who use opioids for genuine medical problems, addiction is rare in RLS patients. Addiction includes a number of specific phenomena, such as dependence – need of the medication to maintain a comfortable, normal state; tolerance, decreased responsiveness to a given dose that leads to escalating doses; and drug-seeking behaviors. In my experience, patients using opioids do show gradual increase in the dose required, but rarely show the dependence and drug-seeking behaviors that are so evident in the usual addiction. Even dependence, which means there are uncomfortable sensations when the drug is withdrawn, may be acceptable for patients with severe RLS who cannot be managed by other medications. And drug-seeking behavior does occur with other medications, such as L-DOPA combinations. Therefore, I feel that, with the exception of patients who have a history of drug-seeking behavior, opioids can be safely used for RLS. Their physical side effects (such as drowsiness, constipation, and urinary retention) and long-term safety profile compares favorably with other primary medications for RLS. The major problem for prescribing these medications may be the physician's imagined or real fear of regulatory disapproval.

Recently, a new medication called tramadol (Ultram) has been introduced for pain. This medication acts like an opioid, but also has some actions similar to anti-depressants such as fluoxetine (Prozac). It is not clear which action is the important one for tramadol or whether both are important. Although no studies have been done as of yet, I have been told anecdotally that some RLS patients have benefited from tramadol. If it turns out to be a successful RLS medication because of its opioid-like actions, it may be quite useful. Since it is not classified as a narcotic, doctors may feel much freer prescribing tramadol for RLS patients than they would opioid medications.

Summary of Primary Medications:

Most patients with RLS will respond, to some degree, to medications of all three primary classes. The dopamine-related medications and opioids, in particular, seem to have substantial benefits for almost all patients, including those who are quite severely affected. The major consideration then, in using these medications, is to find the one or the combination which works best for the individual patient. That's the good news and it truly is good news for RLS patients. The bad news or at least the qualified news is that all these medications must be used cautiously, since they all have some psychoactive side effects, especially in older patients. Moreover, the long-term effects for younger patients consigned to potentially lifetime therapy with these agents is not clear either. Therefore, these medications should not be used indiscriminately or in doses greater than required for satisfactory symptom relief.

Secondary treatment

As mentioned above, secondary treatment is that which has not been well established or whose efficacy is limited. A couple of classes of medications have been suggested to be useful for RLS, but lack the clearly established benefit and general utility established for the primary medications: anticonvulsant medications and medications that operate on the adrenergic system of the brain. Secondary medications may have some specific uses, but in general, most sleep physicians would seem to try them only after primary medications have failed. In addition to the two classes of secondary medications, there are a number of other medications which should be mentioned for potential use.

Anticonvulsant Medications

Anticonvulsants are medications that suppress seizures. They are, therefore, most used in epilepsy. In various publications, three anticonvulsant medications have been reported to be helpful in at least some patients with RLS. Carbamazepine (Tegretol) has been most systematically studied. Valproic acid (Depakene) has been reported to be helpful in some cases and, most recently, gabapentin (Neurontin) has been suggested to be useful for RLS patients. Whether these medications act by similar mechanisms is unknown and whether other anticonvulsants might help other patients is unknown. Usually, the medications are given in doses that approach the normal doses for seizures; carbamazepine, 600 to 1200 mg per day; Valproic acid, 1000 to 3000 mg per day; and gabapentin, 300 to 2700 mg per day. Especially with carbamazepine, there is a fairly narrow therapeutic window, so blood levels must be monitored. In addition, carbamazepine and, to a lesser extent, Valproic acid are known to cause injuries to the white blood cells and liver, so blood monitoring needs to be carried out at least twice a year. The mode of action of these medications is obscure, but, in general, they may be expected to shift the balance between excitation and inhibition in the nervous system. They favor inhibition in some brain cell circuits, thereby reducing the abnormal discharges of epilepsy and perhaps also the abnormal discharges, if such do in fact exist, which underlie RLS symptoms.

Medications acting on the Adrenergic system

The adrenergic system is composed of those cells whose neurotransmitters are adrenalin and noradrenalin. In general, these transmitters act to stimulate and tune up the brain. In the rest of the body, they increase metabolism, the strength of the heart's action, and the tone of blood vessels, raising the blood pressure. These brain chemicals act upon two general kinds of receptors, complex proteins which receive the neurotransmitter message and make sure the receiving cell hears about it. The alpha receptor is most important for raising blood pressure by increasing the tone of blood vessels, while the beta receptor has more effect on the heart. An alpha receptor antagonist, clonidine (Catapres), has been shown in a double blind study to be helpful for RLS, especially for the waking sensory symptoms and related restlessness. Therapeutic doses have typically been in the range of 0.3 to 0.7 milligrams, although some patients have required higher doses. Clonidine therapy must be begun gradually, with an initial dose of 0.1 milligram a night, because there may be a steep initial drop in blood pressure. Clonidine is usually used for the treatment of high blood pressure, but it also has a role in reducing addictive dependence, such as an addiction to nicotine or opioids. Clonidine should never be stopped abruptly, since a rebound in blood pressure can occur. Another alpha-adrenergic blocker, phenoxybenzamine, has been reported to help PLMS.

A beta receptor blocker, propranolol (Inderal), has also been used with some reported success. Beta blockers are used for a wide variety of conditions, from treatment of high blood pressure, to reducing cardiac arrythmias to managing stage fright or aggression in patients with severe brain disease. The dose range here is unclear, but in its usual therapeutic uses, ranges of 40 to 320 milligrams per day are common. Beta blockers are contraindicated in many patients with lung disease such as emphysema, defective conduction in the heart, and should be used cautiously in patients with diabetes. Like clonidine, treatment should be started gradually, perhaps with a 10 milligram tablet, and never discontinued abruptly. Stopping beta blockers abruptly can lead to serious damage to the heart. Propranolol is available in an extended release form. There are a wide variety of other beta blockers, some of which are better tolerated by patients with lung disease, but these have not been reported to be used in RLS.

Miscellaneous Secondary Medications

Baclofen (Lioresal), an anti-spastic agent, was studied as therapy for PLMS. It was found to improve sleep, but not the actual number of PLMS. Like the benzodiazepines, it acts upon the GABA system of the brain, the neurotransmitter system that is involved in sending an inhibitory or quieting message to the target brain cells. It is usually used to treat abnormal spasms, particularly those that occur in spinal cord disease or multiple sclerosis, as well as some pain syndromes due to problems in a particular nerve. Doses used range from about 20 to 100 milligrams per day.

The following medications have not been formally studied and all reports, even those which have been published, are anecdotal. I mention them here for completeness and as possible last-ditch medications that could be considered if none of the others has worked.

Sedative medications, other than the benzodiazepines, can be considered for RLS. For example, barbiturates such as phenobarbital might be useful. Mysoline, an anticonvulsant that is converted into phenobarbital, is another possibility. Even alcohol has been mentioned as possibly helpful. Since alcohol in moderation can promote health, an aperitif or two might be a good way to begin a dinner party and also relieve RLS that might be provoked by sitting at a table for several hours. Of course, the side effects of sedatives, including alcohol, must be kept in mind, especially drowsiness and dependence. In addition, alcohol puts us to sleep initially, but tends to wake us up in the middle of the night.

Analgesics, other than opioids, have also been reported by various patients to be helpful. Perhaps aspirin and acetaminophen (Tylenol) have been most commonly noted as helpful, although other non-steroidal anti-inflammatory drugs (NSAIDs) such as ibuprofen

(Motrin) or piroxicam (Feldene), might work as well. Usually, one or two pills are taken in the evening.

Some patients also feel that antidepressants, either tricyclic antidepressants such as amitryptiline (Elavil) or serotonin re-uptake blockers (SRUPs) such as fluoxetine (Prozac), have given them relief. Some physicians feel that quinine sulfate, often used for cramps, may help RLS.

Symptomatic Treatment

When RLS or PLMS are due to underlying disorders, treatment of the underlying condition may alleviate the RLS and PLMS. This has not been generally well studied. An alternative is to use standard RLS therapy, as has been studied in kidney failure (uremia) patients. Their RLS has been reported to respond to benzodiazepines, dopaminergic agents, opioids, and clonidine. Dialysis, in particular, can be very challenging for patients with RLS, since they are kept confined and expected to lie still for several hours. Therapy can be tailored around the dialysis session. Where RLS is provoked by a pinched nerve in the back (radiculopathy), proper treatment such a surgery may relieve the associated RLS.

Deficiency states in which the body lacks a required nutrient such as a certain vitamin might be corrected. This has been shown by uncontrolled trials to be true with iron supplementation in iron deficiency and reported for transfusion in anemia. One group has linked folate deficiency to RLS and found improvement of RLS along with other symptoms with treatment. Other treatments, including a number of vitamins, such as vitamin C, vitamin E, or B_{12} are more speculatively linked to deficiency. I am aware of no controlled trials demonstrating that these therapies are effective, although there are suggestive clinical reports.

Medications and other Substances to Avoid

Among the medications that have been suggested to increase RLS or PLMS are the major tranquilizers, called neuroleptics, which are used to treat serious psychiatric disorders. Among these medications are chlorpromazine (Thorazine), haloperidol (Haldol), and fluphen-azine (Mellaril). All of these neuroleptics act, to some extent, to reduce activity in the dopamine system of the brain. It is easy to see, therefore, why they might bother patients with RLS who are so often benefited by dopamine-related medication. Neuroleptics also cause a condition of restlessness which, in some respects, resembles RLS and is called akathisia (which means, in essence, restlessness). In fact, RLS and akathisia (often called neuroleptic induced akathisia, or NIA, to note its connection to the neuroleptics) are sometimes both called restless legs, which can be confusing. Indeed, they do respond, in some cases, to the same medications, such as beta blockers and opioids but they have some distinct features as well. RLS patients are bothered by uncomfortable sensations, by rest, and by evening and night, whereas akathisia patients complain more about a general urge to move and often feel just as uncomfortable when they are standing or at all different times of the day. In addition to neuroleptics, other medications that block the dopamine system, such as the medication metoclopramide (Reglan), which is taken to prevent stomach irritation, can cause akathisia. Probably, any medication that causes akathisia should be avoided by patients with RLS. Akathisia can occur without medication exposure, but it is much rarer.

Other psychiatric medications can also cause problems for RLS patients. It has been fairly often reported that tricyclic antidepressants, such as amitryptilene (Elavil), can make PLMS worse. Other antidepressants are also suspect. Paradoxically, some patients find that these medication can make their RLS symptoms better. Given their problematic nature, however, they are probably best avoided.

Caffeine may also play a dual role in RLS. Its stimulant, alerting properties, reducing the relaxed state, may actually improve RLS symptoms transiently. A number of patients find that this can provide significant relief. However, caffeine can also disrupt sleep, even when taken early in the day, and may provoke a withdrawal syndrome in which RLS symptoms return, perhaps even with a vengeance. Many doctors treating RLS feel it can be useful for RLS patients to reduce caffeine intake.

Nonpharmacologic therapies

A number of nonpharmacological therapies have been suggested for RLS. These have generally been proposed on the basis of case studies or small non-blinded trials. One such therapy is the use of transdermal stimulation. In this technique, a small electric current is passed into the skin. By setting up a competing sensory stimulus, it may counteract the sensations of RLS. It is typically used for chronic pain conditions, which, in some ways, do resemble RLS. Since a variety of sensory inputs, e.g., massage, hot showers, or cold packs, can relieve RLS symptoms for some patients, this kind of therapy has an intuitive appeal. Another therapy that has been reported is thermal feedback, a behavioral technique that can increase blood flow to the legs. A basis for the thermal feedback is the suggestion that PLMS may be associated with decreased blood flow to the legs and cold feet. We probably need to try more of such therapies, which can be quite benign and, in the long run, inexpensive, since medications do have drawbacks. What is needed, however, for general acceptance, is the willingness of practitioners to do formal studies of these techniques.

Wayne A. Hening, M.D., Ph.D.
Department of Neurology
Robert Wood Johnson Medical School
University of Medicine and Dentistry of New Jersey
New Brunswick, New Jersey

Chapter Four

Overall Treatment Strategies for Physicians
Wayne A. Hening, M.D., Ph.D.

Putting the treatment together

In earlier chapters, I discussed how a patient and doctor can work together to treat RLS and the various types of medications which have been considered useful in RLS. In this chapter, I review some overall treatment strategies. How does a doctor put it all together? These strategies give some insights into how someone with experience in RLS approaches the treatment of a new patient: when is therapy started? what is the first drug to try, and what happens if that drug doesn't work? What do you do for the patient who seems unable to respond to the normal approaches? I will first share some of the responses that I received to a questionnaire study of RLS treatment that was supported by the Clemente Foundation. Then I will discuss two approaches to the treatment of RLS, the approach used at the Johns Hopkins Sleep Center by Drs. Richard Allen, David Buchholz, and Christopher Earley, and my own treatment approach.

The Clemente Foundation RLS Therapy Questionnaire Study

With the support of the Clemente Foundation, I collected the replies of 29 experts in RLS and sleep disorders who completed a questionnaire on the therapy of RLS. These responses were gathered between May 1994 and May 1995. The doctors who responded estimated that they have collectively treated 2,978 patients with RLS.

Most doctors felt that drug treatments of RLS should be recommended when the RLS is having a notable impact on the patient's quality of life. Therefore, RLS does not always require treatment with medications, especially every day treatment. Many of the doctors also explicitly consider patient preference as quite important in making their recommendation: therapy is initiated when the patient feels it is needed.

The doctors were divided on what they considered the best initial treatment. The favored treatment was L-DOPA, combined with carbidopa, either in the regular (Sinemet) or sustained release form (Sinemet CR). The second favored initial treatment was clonazepam. However, almost all have used on some occasion each of the primary drug classes: benzodiazepines (28 of 29 doctors), dopaminergic agents (27 doctors) opioids, (24 doctors). Twenty-two doctors would use combination therapy, which is simultaneous use of drugs from different primary classes. The doctors used fairly wide ranges of each of the most commonly recommended medications: L-DOPA combined with carbidopa, regular release (100-400 mg of L-DOPA typical, 2,000 mg maximum) or sustained release (200 to 600 mg of L-DOPA, 1,000 mg maximum); pergolide (0.07 - 0.30 mg, 1.3 mg maximum); clonazepam (0.5 - 2.0 mg, 4.0 mg maximum); and codeine (30 - 90 mg, 120 mg maximum).

Major side effects that the doctors reported occurring in some patients included: for L-DOPA combined with carbidopa, GI discomfort, rebound and augmentation; for pergolide, GI discomfort and dizziness; for clonazepam, sedation, fatigue and confusion; and for opioids, constipation and sedation. Other medications used by three or more of the respondents included: iron, baclofen, vitamins, clonidine, carbamazepine and anticonvulsants.

The Hopkins approach

The Hopkins Sleep Center team (in an approach developed by Richard Allen, David Buchholz, and Christopher Early) makes an initial clinical diagnosis of RLS, excluding secondary causes that may require symptomatic therapy. They then recommend an overnight sleep recording, polysomnogram (PSG), for confirmation of diagnosis and determination of the pattern of PLMS. The PSG can also help determine whether other sleep disorders in addition to RLS, such as sleep apnea, are present. These conditions do not usually respond to the normal RLS medications. They have also found that unless a typical PLMS pattern associated with RLS is present (that is, that most PLMS occur in the first third of the night), therapy is also difficult with standard medications.

Recently the Hopkins Group began to use different initial treatments for RLS, depending on the nature of the patient's disorder. For mild cases of RLS, in which the symptoms are confined to the late evening around bedtime and early in the night, they begin treament with low dose L-DOPA combined with carbidopa (25/100 mg), beginning with half a tablet before bedtime and then increasing as needed by 1/2 tablet every three days until symptoms early in the night are suppressed. If regular L-DOPA combined with carbidopa is inadequate or causes problems, they switch the patient to the sustained-release combination.

Because many patients on L-DOPA will develop rebound of symptoms late in the sleep period or augmentation of symptoms appearing earlier in the day than before treatment, it may be necessary to switch patients to another agent. The first choice for this medication is pergolide which alleviates the problems for most patients. Almost all patients, in their experience, respond initially to these dopaminergic medications. If patients have no response, they feel that it usually means there is some other contributing sleep disorder besides RLS.

Patients who have severe RLS when first seen, especially those with symptoms throughout the night or during the daytime, will almost inevitably require multiple doses of L-DOPA combined with carbidopa and high dose levels. The Hopkins group now feels that almost all of these patients will shortly develop rebound and augmentation and so now will begin their therapy with pergolide, skipping L-DOPA. As in other cases, however, pergolide is begun slowly and gradually increased.

When patients have failed or cannot tolerate the dopaminergic agents, they will give opioids or benzodiazepines, either alone or together with a dopaminergic agent. For truly refractory cases, a strong opioid like levodromoran may prove useful. In their hands, most secondary medications have not been helpful. However, they have recently been giving patients gabapentin (Neurontin). They find that approximately one third of patients have a good response and that almost all of these experience their leg discomforts as actually painful. This subgroup of patients with actual pain might be considered for early trials of gabapentin.

My personal views

I believe in treating RLS patients when their symptoms are bothersome and cannot be managed by the tricks or routines which patients often use to quiet their legs. These include hot baths, massages, avoiding caffeine or other problematic medications, or a bit of appropriately-timed exercise. I believe in treating periodic limb movement disorder (PLMD) patients when their movements appear to be the sole or an important cause of disturbed sleep that bothers them. I will treat RLS patients without polysomnography but, at least for now, only polysomnography can diagnose PLMD. Polysomnography can be useful in RLS to rule out coexisting disorders and determine the degree of sleep disruption caused by RLS (primarily, difficulty in getting to sleep) and related PLMS. In the future, many of these tests may be carried out with monitoring in the patient's own home, reducing the cost and the inconvenience of a sleep study.

Therapy is initiated with medications tailored to the patients' symptoms:

1. If the patient has complaints primarily of sleep dysfunction and daytime somnolence, my initial choice for therapy is a benzo-

diazepine, such as clonazepam or temazepam. This would be the case if the patients had PLMS alone. The initial dose of clonazepam would be 0.5 mg, increased as necessary to 2 mg; of temazepam, 15 mg increased to 30 mg if necessary. If those failed, I would add a dopaminergic agent.

2. If the patient has primarily waking complaints, I would consider either a mild opioid such as propoxyphene (Darvon) or a dopaminergic agent. I have had good experiences with bromocriptine (Parlodel) as an initial agent, beginning with 2. 5 mg at bedtime and increasing to 10 to 20 mg in divided doses. L-DOPA combined with carbidopa, like the opioids, is useful when given in a single shot for symptoms that occur at specific times (e.g., during travel or during public functions). Pergolide has been helpful for some patients in doses ranging from 0.1 to 1.5 mg per day.

3. After therapy is initiated, dose level is tailored to the patient's needs, as is the timing of the individual doses. I try to use as little medication as possible. It is to be expected that, over time, opioid doses may increase. I am reluctant to give L-DOPA combined with carbidopa around the clock. Instead, if a patient had symptoms at times other than the evening and nighttime hours, I would switch to a dopamine agonist, either bromocriptine or pergolide, or to an opioid.

4. Refractory cases have to be judiciously managed by increasing doses, switching primary medications or using combination therapy. Patients often do well on a combination of a dopaminergic agent or opioid for daytime symptoms with a benzodiazepine at night. The worst cases may require triple therapy of opioid, dopaminergic agent, and benzodiazepine. Truly refractory cases have responded to a long-acting opioid such as methadone. I have not tried continuously switching or alternating medications, although others have recommended it. My feeling is that such a regime is a bit too complicated.

5. I use other medications sparingly. Patients with mild symptoms might try vitamin E therapy. If there is iron deficiency, I use iron. Patients intolerant or for some reason unable to use the primary therapeutic classes are then candidates for secondary medications. I

have rarely found these to be helpful, although I have had some patients who responded to propranolol (Inderal) or gabapentin (Neurontin). One patient reported a transient response to fluoxetine (Prozac).

Wayne A. Hening, M.D., Ph.D.
Department of Neurology
Robert Wood Johnson Medical School
University of Medicine and Dentistry of New Jersey
New Brunswick, New Jersey

Author's note: Dr. Hening has shared this medical advice for those physicians who may be unfamiliar with the treatment of RLS. The RLS Foundation, the author and Galaxy Books offer this for informational purposes only.

Chapter Five

Alternative Treatments

---

by Virginia N. Wilson
Ralph Pascualy, M.D., contributor
Alan Kanter, M.D., contributor

Frequently the RLS Foundation office receives a letter telling of a personal experience with a "cure" that completely took the RLS away, and the next day a letter will come to our office saying that same food or vitamin or whatever brings on RLS attacks. For each writer the perfect answer has been discovered, but until a "cure" has been tested over and over again under scientific regulations it cannot be recommended by the Foundation. This is not to say that these are not valid statements of truth. Many cases of RLS have simply disappeared as if by magic. A number of Night Walkers have experienced this miracle, and I wish that every one of us could have that happen. However, often days, months or even years later the RLS reappears. That wily Sleep Thief slips back into the lives of too many.

Dr. Ralph Pascualy, Medical Director of the Providence Sleep Disorders Center in Seattle, said it well in his January 15, 1994, talk before the Seattle RLS group:

> There is a very long list of drugs, treatments, and natural substances that people with restless legs have sworn by. They have said, "My restless legs were cured by this . . . ," or "My restless legs disappeared when I stopped this or that." And we're very puzzled when we try these remedies on other people and they're totally ineffective. Yet we'll have one or two patients who very clearly have the problem found that a calcium pill and potassium supplement, or getting rid of something in their diet did the job. Then a number of people hear about it, do all the same things, and there's absolutely no benefit. There's an old saying that when a lot of things help a condition, probably none of the treatments is very good. I would caution the restless legs community: There is going to be a lot of fanfare and a lot of word of mouth about this or that treatment. Be careful. Certainly, if it's not harmful, try it; but a part of the RLS problem is that many things affect it. One thing we do know is that restless legs come and go. It gets worse and then it gets somewhat better. If you start a treatment, right at the time that you're getting better, you're likely to swear for a least several weeks or months that you were cured by that treatment. If every time that you wear a red tie, it rains, you start thinking, "I need some rain today so I'm going to get out my red tie," even though a part of you knows that's crazy. I think this often happens with restless legs. We need not have closed minds to new treatments, but we need to be careful about our enthusiasm when things are espoused on anecdotal evidence.

We are delighted to receive these letters and the exciting reports of "cures" but since they have not been tested and proved true by clinical trials they must, as Dr. Pascualy cautions, be listed as possible alternative treatments until a later date when they may be evaluated with rigid testing of the research labs. This is not to say that these suggestions are false; the future may prove them to be valuable alternatives to the present medical research which seems to concentrate on pharmaceutical remedies. Physicians in England appear to accept treatment by holistic therapy more than American medical practitioners. The search for proper medications will continue until the cause of RLS has been found. Then a cure may follow.

The following alternative treatments are not endorsed by the RLS Foundation Medical Advisory Board but are offered as possible alternatives to pharmaceutical therapy. Please consult your doctor before trying anything suggested by our well-meaning Night Walkers. The purpose of this book is to enlighten the medical world and the general public about the world of RLS. We do not promise a cure. When someone states the finding of a "cure" we are dubious because as far as we know now, there is none. But if we can help someone find a new way to make living with RLS easier, to help cope with this irritating disorder, we will have achieved our purpose.

● Neuromuscular massage therapy:

Deep muscle massage may be helpful in the case of 'abused' leg muscles (See Section V, Chapter 3, Stop Muscle Abuse). Many RLS victims tend to over-exercise or over-use leg muscles, especially if they are very tired from the constant, unrelenting need to walk and move about. Statements like, "I ride my stationary bike as fast and hard as I can," or "I'd like to beat my legs to a pulp," or "I'd like to cut my legs off with a buzz saw" give cause for concern that muscles are being abused. It has been proposed that the blood vessels and nerves can get trapped in hardened, stressed muscles and unless that pressure is relieved localized anemia (due to the obstruction of the enflow of arterial blood) may result. Often deep massage is painful but rewarding for the relief if affords. There are a number of methods used by therapists, including St. John, Swedish, and Japanese *shiatsu.* A prospective client should check into the quality of the training received. In a newspaper interview massage therapist Brenda

Star Walker states, "A big part is teaching them [her clients] how to help themselves. Five minutes stretching in the morning works wonders. Eating and resting better, paying attention to your body. Plus, it's really therapeutic to rub on a place that hurts. Muscles are like sponges. They get tight, and you rub out toxins including lactic acid. And people long for an hour's worth of time out, because touch is healing." (*Florida Times-Union*, Jan. 28, 1993, p. C-4)

● Sclerotherapy:

Alan Kanter, M.D., of the Vein Center of Orange County, Irvine, California, has been working with the Sleep Disorders Center of the University of California-Irvine. (Kanter, 1995) The total results of his ongoing research are not yet available so it is not possible for us to give an unconditional nod to his work as an effective treatment for RLS, but we asked Dr. Kanter to explain some of his research terminology here.

> Recent evidence suggests that some people with RLS who have coexisting varicose or spider leg veins may find that their RLS symptoms improve after treatment of their vein condition by "sclerotherapy." Although symptoms may recur gradually over time, re-treatment of recurrent veins is thought to bring further improvement in RLS symptoms.

> Sclerotherapy is a century-old non-surgical method of eliminating varicose veins, more commonly practiced in Europe, and currently enjoying renewed popularity in the United States. Intravenous injections of a solution directly into the abnormal veins initiate an inflammatory response resulting in shrinkage and eventual reabsorption of the veins. Treatment usually is done over several sessions as an out-patient procedure, and may involve the use of ultrasound imaging to precisely guide injections to deeper, invisible problem veins.

> It is postulated that microcirculatory changes induced by the abnormal flow in diseased veins stimulates nerve fibers, perceived by the brain as restlessness. Recently published studies in the field

of phlebology have also shown a deficiency in certain nerve fiber transmission ("alpha-adrenergic" and "C-fibre") in the legs of patients with varicose veins.

Properly fitted support hosiery has been shown to alleviate symptoms of venous insufficiency. Since it appears that RLS and leg vein disease may have a common connection, wearing such support hosiery may provide relief to some RLS sufferers. Some warnings are in order. Non-prescription, over-the-counter support hose may aggravate the problem, and should generally be avoided. Higher quality hosiery (sometimes known as surgical or post-operative weight) is usually prescribed by a doctor after custom fitting, and should be "20-30"or "30-40"graduated strength.

Bulging varicose veins are usually hard to miss. But, because phlebology is several steps behind the field of sleep disorders medicine in fighting the same uphill battle for medical education and recognition, finding a qualified, knowledgeable vein specialist in the U.S. who can recognize more subtle vein disease can be difficult. Clues that you have received a thorough exam include the use of a hand-held portable Doppler device to listen for vein flow patterns of deeper invisible veins in the standing position, and a purposeful exam of all sides of your legs under good lighting while lying on an exam table. Even though you may receive a proper exam, don't count on a vein specialist knowing about RLS and its connections to vein disease. The same applies to sleep disorders specialists; most will not have heard of this connection either.

● Mechanical and electrical massage equipment:

Many tell us that the use of a mechanical or electrical vibrator is helpful in relieving annoying RLS symptoms. There is some evidence for this from the medical literature.

● Vitamins, herbs, and diets:

• Vitamin E

This vitamin seems to have the most proponents. In looking for documented research of this therapy we found very little printed material in reliable medical journals. This could be due either to the lack of controlled research on the subject or a biased viewpoint against simplistic treatments by American medically-accepted journals. Two dermatologists happened upon the discovery that patients using vitamin E capsules of 400 international units, one to three times a day before meals, remarked about the cessation of "jumping legs." After describing nine restless legs cases with positive help from the vitamin therapy, the author concludes his article saying:

> Our interest in muscle spasms arose as the result of what might be called a beneficial side-effect of vitamin E which we were prescribing for completely unrelated dermatological conditions. The problem of the "restless legs" syndrome belongs in the field of internal medicine or orthopedic surgery and it is to be hoped that someone with access to more patients with this condition will launch a large-scale investigation into the patho-physiology of the condition and the reason vitamin E controls it. We are merely calling attention to a simple effective, innocuous treatment for a serious therapeutic problem. (Ayers et al., 1973)

• Vitamin B

A German-trained nurse from Hartford, Connecticut, and a number of other Night Walkers believe that vitamin B elements are helpful and need to be included in the diet daily as long as the patient lives. [This might be true if the patient were tested deficient in vitamin B which includes the elements, B_1, B_6, and B_{12} (thiamine, pyridoxine, and riboflavin).]

• Folate (folic acid, a vitamin of the B complex)

Folate deficiency in pregnant women tends to exacerbate the condition of restless legs (Botez, 1994) and may be a cause for the prominence of the disorder among the low-income elderly. Researchers found that 60% of senior citizens tested in the Miami area had folate levels below normal. Folate may be found in leafy green vegetables – spinach, beet greens, and kale. Liver and kidney also provide excellent amounts of the nutrient. Caution: folate is easily destroyed by over-cooking. Quick steaming is recommended. (Alan R. Gaby, M.D., Pikesville, Maryland – personal communication)

"One study shows a familial form of restless legs syndrome responds to large doses of folic acid, such as 10 mg per day." ("Food and Nutrition," *Prevention*, 1993)

• Iron

K. A. Ekbom (1960) did some serious but uncontrolled research into iron deficiency and RLS and then he treated patients with iron. This note and a news clipping sent by a Night Walker of Escondido, California, may be an echo to this study: "Make sure you're getting enough iron. Restless leg syndrome has long been associated with iron-deficiency anemia. Older people who are taking drugs for arthritis may have a low iron status." (Alan R. Gaby, M.D., Pikesville, Maryland – personal communication)

• Magnesium

There is recent evidence from the literature that RLS patients may be deficient in magnesium.

• Multivitamins

Health experts keep reminding all of us that it is important to watch our diets and our vitamin intake every day. Keeping healthy is most important for the RLS sufferer, as the energy produced in the body each day is drained and needs to be replenished. Vitamins, diet, and exercise unite as a team to help Night Walkers cope.

• Herbs

Herb culturist Louise Allen of Findlay, Ohio, writes that a surprising new interest has emerged: the medicinal side of aromatic herbs.

I know that even during worst RLS flare-ups and after night walking I put three drops of the lavender on a tissue or pillow and it's reminiscent of my childhood aches and pains with mother's comforting presence. It is said that one is drawn to the fragrance the body needs most. The olfactory nerve (sense of smell) is connected directly to the limbic section of the brain where pleasures (emotion and motivation) are experienced.

Most commonly clary sage is used to ease depression, as is ylang ylang. Many use it to alleviate anger. To ease mental stress, anxiety, and nervousness, Chamomile and lavender. To me lavender is the most soothing. Put these under the edge of the pillow slip, next to the head and savor the aromatic pleasure. Sometimes sleep will follow. **One must remember that these aromatic herbs are drug plants to aid rest only. They are not to be taken internally.**

• Red wine

We had a number of letters, including some from physicians themselves, saying that a glass of red wine before retiring aided in getting to sleep. The RLSF Medical Advisory Board does not recommend alcohol for sleep disorders since scientific studies have shown that it may improve sleep for the first half of the night but it disrupts sleep during the second half of the night.

As I stated earlier in this chapter, many letters come to us saying certain treatments, herbs, foods, vitamins, or seasonings have eliminated restlessness while others declare that the same things caused the writer's RLS to worsen. We chose not to include these conflicting suggestions and opinions in order not to confuse our readers. But we can assure you that for every positive suggestion, we have had an equal number of opposing opinions. Here is a definitive assessment with which most of us can agree:

The difficulty is that at times the restless legs seem to "do their own thing" no matter what I eat. As a result, it is difficult to determine what food is generally acceptable.   *C. R., Dallas, Texas*

Note: Details of references can be found in Appendix 3, Publications Relating to RLS.

Chapter Six

Questions and Answers from RLS Newsletter September 1993

Answers by Dr. Arthur S. Walters
Chairman of the RLS Foundation Medical Advisory Board

Q. Is there any medicine for RLS other than Sinemet? Any relief other than walking?

A. Levadopa and Carbidopa combined (Sinemet)

Opioids (Darvon, Percocet, Tylenol with Codeine)

Benzodiazepines (Klonopin, Valium)

Clonidine (Catapres)

Carbamazepine (Tegretol)

Baclofen (Lioresal)

Bromocriptine (Parlodel)

Pergolide (Permax)

(Author's note: In 1996 gabapentin [Neurontin] has been added to this list.)

Q. Should Sinemet be taken around the clock? What about dosage of Sinemet? Does it hurt to break in half?

A. Regular Sinemet or long-acting Sinemet CR can be broken in half without loss of efficiency. Consult individual physician regarding around-the-clock use. Dosage must be individualized for each person separately.

Q. Can Sinemet CR be harmful?

A. Most common side effects are nausea and G.I. upset. Occasionally Sinemet may cause temporary involuntary movement like chorea or dystonia in high doses. In high doses it has the potential to cause temporary mental confusion, but I have not seen this yet in RLS.

Q. Is there any way to determine when to take the medication [Sinemet CR], such as 12 hours, 8 hours, 6 hours? What is safe?

A. I usually suggest taking medication at least 45 minutes before the usual onset of symptoms, since it takes that long for it to digest and get into the brain.

Q. Instead of increasing medication is there another drug that I could rotate with Sinemet?   What can I try? I need help!

A. See answer to question one.

Q. What is the best medicine (and what frequency, dosage, and sequence)? My neurologist says Sinemet is the only one that works. Is that true?

A. Sinemet is probably the best drug. Dose has to be individualized for each individual patient. Not true that Sinemet is only drug for RLS, see answer to question one.

Q. Any new drugs available yet?

A. See answer to question one.

Q. Soma helps me sleep in sequence with Sinemet. Is this combination harmful?

A. No, combination not harmful.

Q. Klonopin does not seem to be effective in the daytime. Would a larger dose be helpful?

A. Maybe. Consult a physician. Dosage must be individualized for each patient separately depending on level of therapeutic response and whether patient can tolerate drug without side effects.

Q. Does anyone get hot feet?

A. Yes, but if so, should be checked by physician to rule out peripheral neuropathy.

Q. Most RLS patients have the problem in the legs. Is there anyone like me – crawling in the ankles?

A. Yes.

Q. My neurologist seems to think that people with RLS are born lacking a certain chemical.

A. Could be – which chemical is as yet unknown.

Q. Does stress have a bearing on RLS? Also anxiety?

A. Yes. Any movement disorder can get worse with stress, anxiety.

Q. Is there a relationship between Parkinson's and RLS?

A. Parkinson's patients can also get RLS. This may or not be coincidental or could be related to anti-Parkinson drugs.

Q. I have MS. Is there any relationship between MS and RLS?

A. No definite relationship established at this point.

Q. I've heard RLS is a central nervous system disorder, which seems right to me. I feel it stems from the base of my spine – top of buttocks area. Pressure here relieves spasm.

A. Site of origin of the abnormality in the nervous system of RLS patients is currently unknown. Any counteracting stimulus may give temporary relief of symptoms. Another example of this would be rubbing the legs to get relief.

Q. Why do attacks go from one leg to the other? Never both OK same time.

A. RLS may affect one leg, then the other, or both legs simultaneously. Reason for this is currently unknown.

Q. Does anyone get lasting relief from RLS? Does it get worse as you age?

A. Yes, there are spontaneous remissions, and sometimes the remissions can last indefinitely. Tends to worsen with age, but not always.

Q. I am pregnant. What medications would be safe for me to take for my RLS.?

A. No medication for RLS is considered safe during pregnancy. Consult with your gynecologist.

Q. Wonder if barometer changes have an effect on RLS?

A. Don't know – has not been studied heretofore.

(Author can answer this – for some of us, yes. *Night Walkers* had a research test but didn't have enough willing to participate. Some noticed the *rise or fall* of the barometer increased symptoms. The greatest help to those of us who were bothered is the fact that we realized that we weren't getting worse – just that we couldn't do anything about the weather!)

SECTION III

RLS Around the World

RLS Around the World

The first International Symposium on Restless Legs Syndrome and Related Disorders, held in Florence, Italy, on May 25, 1994, was organized by two members of the RLS Foundation Medical Advisory Board, Drs. Arthur S. Walters and Wayne A. Hening. Since then much interest in RLS has spread throughout the world. The *RLS Newsletter* is mailed to Night Walkers and physicians in nineteen countries including Australia, Belgium, Canada, Czech Republic, England, Finland, Germany, Greece, Israel, Italy, Japan, Mexico, New Zealand, Norway, Peru, Portugal, and Sri Lanka.

SLEEP THIEF is pleased to include several articles written by authors from other nations.

Chapter One

Restless Legs Syndrome: A Historical and Personal Survey

Giorgio Coccagna, M.D. and Elio Lugaresi, M.D.

Wherefore to some, when being abed they betake themselves to sleep, presently in the arms and legs, leapings and contractions of the tendons, and so great a Restlessness and tossing of their members ensue, that the diseased are no more able to sleep, than if they were in a place of the greatest torture.

Th. Willis, 1695

As Critchley reported (1955), the first unequivocal description of Restless Legs Syndrome (RLS) to appear in medical literature was that of the English physician Thomas Willis in 1695. Two centuries were to pass before another report was published by the German doctor Wittmaack (1861) describing a patient with this unusual disorder. Wittmaack considered the complaint to be a form of hysteria and called it *anxietas tibiarum*. Later on, Beard (1880), Bing (1913) and, briefly, Oppenheim (1923) mentioned *anxietas tibiarum* in their writings and it continued to be held a sign of neurosis.

Oppenheim did, however, mention that this form of neurosis could be a familial or hereditary complaint.

In 1936 Code and Allen reported in the Proceedings of the Mayo Clinic three cases of neurosis involving the legs. The second of these reports was probably a case of Restless Legs Syndrome.

The first detailed description of the clinical features of RLS was published by Mussio, Fournier and Rawak in 1940. They pointed out the exacerbating effect of pregnancy and stressed the hereditary and familial nature of the disorder. They also denied the neurotic origin of the disease and postulated a central nervous system impairment. In 1947, they returned to the topic and proposed the more descriptive term of *agitation paresthésique des extrémités* (paresthetic restlessness of the extremities) thus emphasizing that the symptoms could also involve the upper limbs.

In 1943, Allison described the hallmarks of RLS, which he too suffered, under the term "leg jitters" and was the first to note the presence of involuntary muscular jerks. Two years later, it was Ekbom who wrote detailed papers defining all the clinical features of the syndrome to which he gave the name by which it is universally known today. Alongside the classic paresthetic form (*asthenia crurum paresthetica*), he also described a painful form (*asthenia crurum dolorosa*) whose symptoms are not confined to the nocturnal hours and are not accompanied by an urgent need to move the legs and feet.

Since Ekbom, further reports from the French school have added to our knowledge of RLS (Bonduelle and Jolivet 1947-53). These authors implicated a circulatory disturbance in the lumbar spine consisting in slowing of venous flow triggered by decubitus (bed sores) or by pregnancy as the origin of RLS.

After Allison's first report, the only studies explicitly referring to the presence of involuntary muscular jerks accompanying the motor restlessness during sleep were those of the Italian Tuvo (1949) and the Israeli Bornstein (1961). Bornstein also postulated that the complaint was caused by a defect in muscular tone regulation due to an impairment of the descending reticular substance of the nervous system with secondary effects on the gamma component of the nervous system at the level of the spinal cord.

When we first encountered a case of RLS in 1962, we found ourselves, like many neurologists and virtually all general practitioners, wholly unaware of the existence of this syndrome. We were perplexed to find ourselves confronted by a friar who had been admitted to our ward that morning. He gave us an exasperated account of how he had been tormented for a lifetime by an indescribable sensation in his legs which would start in the evening whenever he sat down and above all when he went to bed. He would be overcome by an irresistible urge to move his legs frenetically and was almost always forced to get up and run or jump about the room. Only in the early morning hours would the disorder subside, leaving him exhausted.

From the look on our faces, the poor friar was disappointed to find that yet again, whenever he decided to consult a specialist, after blood tests and a thorough investigation of muscles and nerves, the conclusion would be that he had a psychosomatic complaint which manifested itself in the lower limbs. In vain would he protest that he was the calmest man in the world, he had embraced his religious life with enthusiasm and had never regretted his decision, he was at peace with the world and his faith was unshakable despite the torment wrought upon him each night by the devil. His fellow friars had become resigned to the fact that one of their fellows was somewhat strange, and after yet another hospital admission, they would have treated him with even greater suspicion and diffidence.

This time, be it by chance or by luck, things went differently. After a few days, when events were moving in the direction the friar had predicted, one of us remembered having read in the journal *Neurology* an article by a Swede by the name of Ekbom who described a clinical picture similar to that presented by the friar.

Having confirmed this, we began to take things very seriously indeed. Since we had already begun to take an interest in sleep disorders, we decided that the first thing to do was to document the type of insomnia accompanying this syndrome.

At that time, our sleep laboratory had only a rudimentary set of equipment and no technicians. The neurologist had to supervise all-night recordings himself after a nurse had helped him position the electrodes on the patient's scalp, chin and eyes' outer contour. This do-it-yourself situation proved fortunate, because during the night the doctor following the recording, separated from the patient only by a screen, was so impressed by the frenetic leg movements that he decided to attach two electrodes to the anterior tibialis muscles of the legs as well.

For the first part of the night the tracing was full of artifacts produced by the jumping pens, then suddenly everything calmed down and the first signs of sleep appeared on the electroencephalogram (EEG). The doctor, sitting comfortably in an armchair was about to follow the friar into the land of Morpheus, when he heard an intermittent rustling in the room. After a minute or so, he realized that the noise was produced by the pens connected to the tibialis muscles. There was no doubt that the friar was sleeping because wide clear-cut K complexes were being drawn on the EEG tracing. The doctor peeped behind the screen to check that this was truly the case, when he noticed that the friar's legs underneath the covers would suddenly bend every 20-25 seconds and then resume the normal position. This went on throughout the recording except for one stage of slow-wave sleep (deep sleep). During a rapid eye movement sleep or dream sleep (REM) episode the movements would disappear, but they persisted, less intensely during a subsequent REM stage. When the ward neurologists were shown the tracing on the following morning, they had to admit that they were dealing with something they had never seen before.

Gripped with enthusiasm, we performed another five consecutive nocturnal polygraphic recordings. They were all identical and we were convinced that our patient had a special form of RLS. When the friar realized that someone had finally taken him seriously, he became very cooperative and told us that his mother and a couple of his eight brothers and sisters whom he seldom saw had or had had a very similar disorder. The search for the Tassoni family was on: six of his brothers were examined directly by us, another two who had emigrated, were contacted by mail. All of them recounted a typical history of RLS and also confirmed that their mother, who in the meantime had died, had suffered from a severe form of a similar disorder. Three brothers agreed to undergo one or more nocturnal polygraphic recordings and thus it was that we were pleased to find that they too presented a nocturnal polygraphic picture identical to that of their brother, the friar: rhythmic muscular jerks recurring for most of the night, mainly during light sleep, but sometimes persisting in deep slow-wave sleep and REM sleep. The only remaining doubt was whether this polygraphic picture was typical of that particular family, or the hallmark of sporadic cases of RLS too.

Once we had clarified the clinical features of the syndrome, it was not difficult to track down another ten cases, all of whom were monitored polygraphically. They all presented the periodic muscular jerks during sleep which were recorded on cine-film in some cases. By now it was clear that the jerks were the hallmark of RLS and ruled out a psychogenic origin of the disorder once and for all.

It didn't take much to convince us that RLS must have been one of the commonest disorders on earth: we only had to mention our research and a long line of friends and relatives would join the myriad of patients who experience this torture daily whenever they go to the cinema, theater, relax to watch TV, or retire to bed. One of our wives told us that her dressmaker confessed to having slept the best part of thirty years in an armchair with a blanket over her knees because every 2-3 minutes she would have to get up and walk about the room until the early hours of the morning. Her husband had offered her an ultimatum: either she left the matrimonial bed or he would leave her. Of course, we invited her to our laboratory for a recording, but after an hour of indescribable torment, she had to be released to walk, or rather jump about the room. Another three attempts were made to obtain a recording, but in vain.

Another episode occurred in the mid Sixties when a middle-aged couple were referred to our laboratory. The wife complained that her husband would kick her in bed at meticulously regular intervals for most of the night, disturbing her sleep. The husband said that he was not aware of anything and suspected his fussy wife of exaggerating. The husband underwent polygraphic recording and sure enough he presented rhythmic muscular jerks in the legs for virtually the whole duration of sleep, identical to those observed in RLS. Yet the patient swore that he had never experienced any unpleasant sensation in his limbs.

We thus got into the habit of recording the electromyogram of the anterior tibialis muscles of nearly all patients undergoing polysomnography for one reason or another. We had soon gathered quite a lot of evidence of patients who presented rhythmic leg jerks for much of the night, without ever having experienced pain or discomfort in their legs. These cases were published in 1966 and grouped under the term Nocturnal Myoclonus (NM).This term had been coined by Symonds but it was not really a very appropriate label, as Symonds had described a wide and varied group of motor phenomena occurring in sleep predominated by benign and non repetitive body jerks at sleep onset, sometimes accompanied by hallucinations (hypnagogic hallucinations) and sensory shocks. The report also included a typical case of familial RLS. Symonds postulated an epileptic origin for these myoclonic jerks (myo=muscle; clonic=jerks).

We subsequently collected a number of symptomatic cases of RLS and NM accompanying myelopathy and radiculopathies (disorders of the spinal cord and nerve roots). The term Nocturnal Myoclonus has now been replaced by Periodic Limb Movements in Sleep (PLMS) because the muscular jerks last longer than a normal positive myoclonus which is usually very fast.

Although it was obvious that NM could also occur without the abnormal skin sensations and motor restlessness, we were convinced that the two disorders shared a common origin. In fact, we soon noted that treatments could relieve the limb discomfort, but the nightly jerks would persist. In one case of RLS associated with sleep apnea syndrome, tracheostomy (an old treatment for sleep apnea where an artificial airway was built surgically) resolved the sleep apnea syndrome and got rid of the tingling sensation, but the jerks persisted throughout all sleep stages.

When we saw the first cases of RLS we tried the same treatments suggested by Ekbom and the French authors: vasodilators (blood vessel dilators), barbiturates and drugs acting on the autonomic nervous system. Results were disappointing. Only one drug gave good results in three patients, but treatment had to be suspended sooner or later because of side effects. When we decided to try giving patients Valium, we were happy to find that almost all of them benefitted. The only drawback was that at high doses the drug increased weakness of the leg muscles during the day, a disorder already common in RLS patients. We then found that the beneficial effects of Valium wore off as time passed. We were mulling over alternative therapies when a physician friend who had a severe form of RLS proudly announced that he had solved the problem with baclofen (Lioresal). We offered our patients a similar course of treatment and in 1978 the encouraging results led us to propose this drug as an alternative treatment for RLS.

In the early Seventies the Bologna school had completed the clinical definition and neurophysiology of RLS and suggested treatments which remain valid today. In the following years we performed several electrophysiological studies demonstrating that in both RLS and PLMS there is an impaired excitability curve for the

H reflex (a spinal cord reflex), more marked during the night, with a slope similar to those observed in patients with spasticity. In the light of these findings, it is no surprise to learn that we had already noted in our first patients examined in the Sixties that Babinski's sign was common in the evening hours in patients with RLS. This sign found on physical examination is also found in patients with spasticity. In addition, cine-films and video recordings showed that during the periodic limb movements there is a dorsiflexion (upgoing movement) of the big toe with spreading of the smaller toes, similar to the movements of a Babinski sign. All these findings provide additional evidence for a central nervous system disorder in patients with PLMS and/or RLS.

Unfortunately, our findings, published in minor journals, were ignored by Anglo-Saxon researchers for over ten years. It was only in the Eighties that experts like Mardsen, Thorpy, Walters, and Hening saved our work from oblivion and invited us to present our results at international meetings, in monographs, and books.

Dr. Walters' enthusiasm led him to set up an international RLS study group and he invited us to get in touch with the Tassoni family of old. This family with others all over the world, was to take part in a genetic study to confirm the hypothesis of a likely autosomal dominant mode of inheritance.

We were doubtful that after thirty years we would manage to track down all the family members or even some of them. But luck was on our side yet again. The old friar was very ill, but alive and living only 300 metres from our Clinic. Still grateful for what we had done to help him and his brothers, he made every effort to contact his large family. Within the space of a few weeks we had blood samples from the whole family including the children and grandchildren who had been born in the meantime.

If the ongoing linkage studies are successful, further progress will have been made in characterizing these syndromes. Another step forward will be achieved when we discover the cause of RLS and, above all, when we finally find a cure. Needless to say, this is the achievement long awaited by RLS sufferers who nightly experience the torment of their complaint and for whom the only drugs currently available offer effective, but only transient, relief.

Giorgio Coccagna, M.D.
Elio Lugaresi, M.D.
Clinica Neurologica
Universitá di Bologna
Bologna, Italy

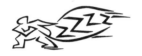

Chapter Two

Restless Legs Syndrome: The Canadian Experience

by Jacques Y. Montplaisir, M.D., Ph.D., FRCP

1.) Restless legs syndrome (RLS): a diagnostic dilemma

a) Clinical diagnosis

In 1977, shortly after returning from California, I opened a sleep disorders center in Montréal. Our research program at that time was to study the neurogenetic, biochemical, and pharmacological aspects of narcolepsy. From the beginning I was impressed by the large number of patients consulting for leg restlessness at bedtime which was associated with a difficulty in falling asleep and multiple nocturnal awakenings.

Although RLS has been known for a long time by some specialists, my early patients had remained undiagnosed on the average for almost twenty years. Several reasons may explain this situation. First, the disease was little known to physicians and even when it was correctly diagnosed, it was often left untreated by clinicians since it does not influence life span or cause invalidity.

Second, patients had difficulty in accurately describing their symptoms – especially the unpleasant sensations associated with leg restlessness. Finally, the diagnosis was also difficult to make because of patient-to-patient differences in symptomatology. Some patients reported mainly leg discomfort or even leg pains without motor restlessness while others reported severe jerking of the legs without any sensory discomfort.

In 1992 we tried to clarify the relationship between sensory and motor symptoms of RLS. We found that in most cases, sensations and movements occur together, but in a substantial number of cases both symptoms may appear independently (Pelletier and Montplaisir, 1992). We therefore concluded that these symptoms should be measured separately when various treatments of RLS are evaluated.

There are many other inter-patient differences in the clinical presentation of RLS (Montplaisir et al., 1996). Some patients have arm discomfort while most patients do not, regardless of RLS severity. In about 40% of patients, symptoms occur predominantly or exclusively on one side (right or left). Most patients experience severe restlessness at bedtime and therefore have sleep-onset insomnia, while others (15%) have no difficulty falling asleep but wake up in the middle of the night with an urge to move. In 20% of patients, symptoms are worse in the summer, while in others there is no seasonal variation. Many patients, but not all, report cravings for food (especially for sugar) when RLS symptoms occur. I remember one patient who gained 80 pounds in one year by eating 10 chocolate bars every night to relieve his RLS symptoms; his nocturnal bulimia subsided and he lost weight after treatment with L-DOPA.

Differences are also seen in response to treatment. This is true especially for opiates. In our experience, one out of five patients treated with opiates shows major improvement. For example, one patient who had more than a thousand leg movements per night before treatment, had only six movements after treatment with codeine. That man did not respond to treatment with L-DOPA although his mother did. Why? And why does the severity of RLS vary so much from patient to patient or throughout a patient's lifetime? The sudden remissions, lasting for months or even years, are as difficult to explain as are the relapses that appear without any apparent reason.

In summary, although RLS is now better known to physicians, several questions about its etiology, psychopathology, and treatment remain unanswered and should be addressed in future research.

b) Sleep laboratory diagnosis

The clinical diagnosis of RLS is at times difficult to make and we have as yet no reliable objective test for it. Due to the lack of objective signs, RLS is often either overlooked by physicians or considered to be a psychosomatic condition. An objective measure of RLS symptoms would serve not only to facilitate diagnosis, but would enhance assessment of various RLS treatments and would certainly speed up the search for a genetic marker.

Most RLS patients also have periodic leg movements during sleep (PLMS), the quantification of which (PLMS index = movements / hour of sleep) is often used to make the diagnosis of RLS. The specificity of this measure has been questioned since PLMS are found in association with several other sleep disorders such as narcolepsy and sleep apnea syndrome. A large number of "non-complaining" subjects also show PLMS – especially with advancing age. In addition, more than 20% of RLS patients, including severe cases, have no PLMS even when recorded for several consecutive nights. For these reasons, we are currently working to develop a test of leg restlessness in the awake patient. Since symptoms are worse at rest and especially in the evening, we designed a test where patients sit motionless on the bed, legs outstretched and eyes open while activity of leg muscles is recorded. This test was called the suggested immobilization test (SIT). Later we modified the test by immobilizing both legs in a stretcher to prevent gross movements of the legs. This modified version of the test was called "the forced immobilization test (FIT)" (Montplaisir et al., 1994b).

In a recent comparative study, we found the SIT superior to the FIT in discriminating RLS patients from normal controls. Several patients reported that they did not contract their leg muscles during the FIT because they knew that the unpleasant sensations would not be relieved by contractions not accompanied by movements. On the other hand, the SIT and the PLMS index were found to be equally able to discriminate patients from normal controls. These two measures, however, were not correlated with each other, suggesting that they assess different components of RLS. More research will be needed to develop a specific and sensitive diagnostic instrument.

2) The prevalence of RLS

The prevalence of RLS was first estimated to be 5% of the general population (Ekbom, 1945). More recently, we conducted a survey through personal interviews across Canada (Lavigne et al., 1994). Of the 2,019 respondents, all over eighteen years of age, 15% reported leg restlessness at bedtime and 10% reported unpleasant leg sensations associated with awakenings during sleep. This survey also showed that RLS-related symptoms increased with age, and were more frequent among French-speaking respondents from Eastern Canada (Lavigne et al., 1994). The presence of a large number of families affected by RLS in the province of Québec may explain these regional differences.

3) Age of onset

RLS is often considered a disease of middle to older age. However, in a recent study of a large number of RLS patients, we found that symptoms appear before age twenty in nearly 40% of patients. Furthermore, we had previously studied a family in which RLS started in the first year of life (Montplaisir et al., 1985). RLS was even documented in a three-year-old child who also showed PLMS in the laboratory. In a recent survey of 2,000 eleven-year-old children, 16.8% reported leg restlessness at bedtime. These results are in agreement with the statement made by Walters and co-workers (Walters et al., 1994), that RLS "may be more common in childhood and adolescence than heretofore recognized."

4) A familial disease

Two thirds of our RLS patients have at least one first-degree relative affected by the condition (Montplaisir et al., 1996). In these families, approximately 40% of all first-degree relatives report symptoms of RLS and in several cases the pedigree suggests an autosomal dominant mode of inheritance.

Eight years ago, we initiated a linkage study to try to localize the RLS gene. For this purpose, we selected one large family where information was available for more than 100 first-degree relatives, 50% of whom were afflicted with RLS. To facilitate interviews and blood collection from relatives, I was invited to attend the 100th anniversary of the family's grandmother, herself afflicted with RLS. With nurses of the Canadian Red Cross, we installed a small stand at the entrance to her country house. Thirty-eight first-degree relatives attended this party. Before entering the house, they all agreed to fill out a questionnaire and to give blood for the genetic study. During the dinner I was invited to give a short talk on RLS to members of the family. I realized there how much RLS symptoms do affect a patient's and, indeed, a family's quality of life.

5) Treatment

In 1985 (Montplaisir et al., 1985), we studied a 36-year-old man (Mr. B.) who, all his life, had unpleasant creeping sensations in both legs that kept him from falling asleep at night and who was awakened every night by involuntary jerks of the legs. A lumbar puncture was performed. Increased levels of dopamine and of homovanillic acid (the main metabolite of dopamine) were found in his cerebrospinal fluid.

Based on this observation, we formulated the hypothesis that RLS and PLMS could be linked to increased dopaminergic activity. Consequently, we treated Mr. B. with gamma-hydroxybutyrate (GHB), a short-acting drug known to block the release of dopamine in the central nervous system. Taken at bedtime, GHB first produced a marked increase in RLS and PLMS symptoms which lasted approximately two hours. This result therefore indicated that, contrary to our initial hypothesis, RLS and PLMS may result from a decrease in central dopaminergic activity. We decided to treat Mr. B. with L-DOPA, the dopamine precursor. This medication produced a suppression of RLS and PLMS for approximately six hours. The patient found this treatment more effective than previous therapeutic trials with clonazepam and baclofen. This first evaluation led us to study the effects of L-DOPA on a larger patient population. In a sleep laboratory study of seven patients, published in 1986 (Montplaisir et al., 1986), we were able to demonstrate the therapeutic value of L-DOPA, a result which was further confirmed by a double-blind placebo-controlled study in 1988 (Brodeur et al., 1994). At that time, we also became aware of a letter which had been published in 1982 (Akpinar, 1982) and in which Dr. Akpinar first reported the therapeutic value of L-DOPA. Since then, L-DOPA has been routinely used to treat RLS. However, as we noted in our 1986 paper (Montplaisir et al., 1986), L-DOPA is a short acting drug and bedtime administration results in movement suppression during the first part of night only, with a rebound of motor restlessness during the last part of the night. More recently, several authors have noted motor restlessness during the day following nighttime administration of L-DOPA. This side effect limits its clinical use. We are now searching for new drugs that are as effective as L-DOPA in treating RLS but that do not produce these undesirable side effects. Several drugs that mimic the effects of dopamine (dopamine agonists) are being developed and there are some indications that they may have major advantages over present treatments.

Studies on dopaminergic drugs and new developments in brain imagery techniques have also opened a new field of research, i.e., the *in vivo* study of dopaminergic function in humans afflicted with RLS. These studies should lead to the discovery of more specific and effective therapeutic approaches.

Jacques Y. Montplaisir, M.D., Ph.D., FRCP
Centre d'etude du Sommeil
Hôpital du Sacré-Coeur
Montréal, Canada

Note: Details of references in text can be found in Appendix 3, Publications Relating to RLS.

Chapter Three

Restless Legs, Your Biological Clock, and You: The Circadian Rhythm of RLS

Arthur S. Walters, M.D.
with
Claudia Trenkwalder, M.D.

Because Restless Legs Syndrome (RLS) is a common, often severe syndrome that is worse at night and results in sleep disturbance, we felt it was important to determine if fluctuations in severity of the RLS symptoms followed the pattern usually seen in a biologically determined 24 hours (circadian) rhythm. Are there hints from the scientific literature that RLS symptoms could follow a circadian rhythm? The answer is yes, most decidedly yes, since sleep itself has a circadian rhythmicity and disruption of that rhythmicity results in sleep disturbance. Let us better understand circadian rhythms, their relation to sleep, and look in more detail at sleep disorders caused by abnormalities of the circadian sleep cycle.

Scientists have discovered that many of our biological functions show daily variations and that the timing of these variations in function can be predicted. For example, it is known that the hormone cortisol is secreted more in the early morning hours and that stomach acid secretion, liver function, white blood cell count, heart and lung function, body temperature, and hunger are all optimum at predictable times of day. All of these entities are also obviously functioning at less than optimum levels at other predictable times of the day. Thus we are better able to utilize certain therapeutic drugs at certain times of the day and we are intellectually sharper at certain times of day; but we are also more susceptible to heart attack and asthma attack in the early morning hours. These predictable fluctuations in bodily functions are called biological rhythms. When these fluctuations occur over approximately a 24 hour period they are called circadian rhythms (circa= about, dies = day – or about a day).

Circadian Rhythms and Sleep

The tendency to be awake during the day and asleep at night is only partly due to the fact that we are most sleepy when we have been awake the longest. Sleep also shows circadian rhythmicity. Core body temperature measurements have traditionally been used as a marker of the circadian sleep cycle. The 24 hour variation in sleep propensity follows the 24 hour variation in body temperature closely and middle to older aged individuals are most drowsy when body temperature is either near its peak at 3 p. m. in the afternoon or when body temperature is near its lowest around 3 a. m. in the morning. Because of this, sleep-deprived drivers are more likely to have auto accidents at these critical times of drowsiness.

The Circadian Biological Clock

Many of our bodily functions that show a 24 hour circadian variation are thought to be controlled by a "biological clock." The biological clock for at least some of these functions is the suprachiasmatic nucleus, a small island of cells in the hypothalamus at the base of the brain. If this clock is surgically removed from the brain in experimental animals, their circadian rhythms are no longer consistent. Some animals have a circadian biological clock that runs somewhat shorter than 24 hours and some animals have a clock that runs somewhat longer than 24 hours. If the suprachiasmatic nucleus from an animal with a different clock time is transplanted into an animal of another type, the receiving animal will then begin to have biological rhythms that fluctuate according to the clock time of the donor animal.

The human circadian biological clock runs closer to 25 hours than 24 hours, but sunlight resets it to 24 hours every morning because bright light causes neural impulses to be transmitted from the eyes to the suprachiasmatic nucleus.

Sleep Disorders Known to Have a Circadian Rhythm Disturbance

Since sleep is regulated by the circadian biological clock, it is not surprising that malfunctions of the clock can lead to sleep disorders.

Delayed sleep phase syndrome

These patients are usually teen-agers and their circadian clock runs late so they go to sleep very late and sleep late. They find it very hard to get up for school.

Advanced sleep phase syndrome

These patients tend to be elderly. Their circadian clock wants to put them to sleep early, so they cannot stay up past dinner and they awaken at 3 or 4 a. m. and cannot go back to sleep.

Non-24 hour syndrome

Some blind individuals have this syndrome. As aforementioned, our circadian clock is closer to 25 hours than 24 hours. In some blind individuals, sunlight cannot reset their clocks to 24 hours so they tend to go to bed later and later and get up later and later. After a while they are sleeping during the day and up all night. Their sleep and wake times will eventually come back to normal times only to again move out of phase.

Irregular sleep wake pattern

These patients have a non-functioning circadian clock and they tend to sleep and to be awake at irregular times. Alzheimer's dementia patients are among those who may suffer from this syndrome.

Some individuals have a normal circadian clock but the environment is out of sync with their clock as in the following examples:

Shift work

Shift workers have to work when their circadian clocks tell them that they should be sleeping and they have to sleep when their clocks tell them they should be awake. Staying awake and staying asleep are both difficult for the shift worker.

Jet lag

People who fly west are tired too early and wake up too early in the new time zone. Those who fly east are not tired when bedtime comes, and they have difficulty getting up in the morning and tend to sleep late in the new time zone.

Does Restless Legs Syndrome Follow a Circadian Rhythm?

Because RLS is characterized by sleep disturbance and is worse at night we wanted to see if there would be a true circadian rhythmicity to the symptoms and to see whether the circadian rhythm would be normal or abnormal as it is in the aforementioned circadian rhythm sleep disorders. Our initial interest in the possible circadian rhythmicity in RLS came from concerns over diagnostic issues which were as follows:

We know for sure that the leg sensations are worse in RLS when patients lie down and the leg sensations are better when patients get up to walk. We know that patients with RLS will have periodic leg movements (PLM) during wakefulness if they are asked to lie very still and that the PLM will also disappear when the patients get up to walk. However, we also know that the leg sensations, restlessness, and PLM are worse at night. **The question can then be asked whether everything is worse at night simply because the patients are lying down more at night or whether there is some other, perhaps circadian, factor that is also making them worse at night.**

To help us answer this question Dr. Claudia Trenkwalder, a visiting fellow from the Max-Planck Institute for Psychiatry in Munich, Germany, came to the laboratory at the Lyons VA Medical Center and the Robert Wood Johnson Medical School where Dr. Wayne Hening and I work.

As you will recall from previous chapters, the major clinical features of RLS are:

a) A desire to move the legs usually associated with discomfort in the legs.

b) Motor Restlessness – patients move to relieve the leg discomfort.

c) The symptoms are worse at rest, i.e., lying or sitting, with at least temporary relief by activity.

d) The symptoms are worse at night.

It was really important to address this issue of circadian rythmicity in RLS because if the symptoms were worse at night simply because patients were lying down more at night, then criteria c) and d) should be collapsed into a single criterion such as "worsening of symptoms at rest, as for example, when lying down at night." If the symptoms got worse at night, not only because patients were lying down, but also because of a circadian factor, then criteria c) and d) should be kept separate. Diagnostic concerns are of obvious importance so that physicians may properly diagnose and treat their patients.

To approach the problem of circadian rhythmicity in RLS we simply subtracted out the "rest factor" criterion c) by having eight volunteers with RLS lie still semi-continuously for three nights and three days in a row. If symptoms still got worse at night, it would most likely be due to a circadian factor and not just because the volunteers were lying down.

We asked the RLS volunteers to rate their leg sensations on a 1-10 scale and we also counted their periodic leg movements **awake and asleep** and then correlated everything to time of day Dr. Trenkwalder dutifully stayed with the patients for three days and our night-time technicians recorded into the wee hours of the morning. We studied eight patients, but three patients from outside the area came to participate in our circadian rhythm project. Carol Walker came to New Jersey courtesy of Dr. June Fry of the Medical College of Pennsylvania and Amelia Lewellen and Kathy Gritton came to us from North Carolina courtesy of the Restless Legs Syndrome Foundation and its Executive Director, Pickett Guthrie.

From the semi-diagrammatic figure (on the chart at the end of the chapter) you can see that for the first two nights and days the leg sensations and PLM were still worse at night even though patients were almost continuously at rest. This suggested that a circadian factor was at work. However, we also realized that several other factors might influence the time of day at which symptoms occurred.

Role of Sleep in RLS

Maybe sleep itself determined the time at which leg sensations, restlessness and PLM occurred during the night and subsequent day. There are plenty of examples of this from the biological literature. For example, some hormones do not follow a circadian rhythm the way cortisol does, but are produced only during sleep no matter what time of day or night the sleep might occur.

To look at this possibility we made the third night of our study a night of total sleep deprivation, but the patients continued to rate their leg sensations and we continued to count their PLM. From the figure you can see that sleep actually plays a negative role since the PLM are a little more pronounced in night three when the patients are kept awake than they are in nights one and two when the patients are asleep. However, the role of sleep is minor since the PLMs are still worse at night than during the day. The sleep deprivation night was also important so that we could get the patients to rate their leg sensations in the middle of the night and, as you can see from the figure, the leg sensations are still worse at night than they are on the preceding or following day. Thus, although sleep plays a role in RLS, it does not seem to alter the shape of the underlying circadian rhythm, i.e., worsening of symptoms at night and amelioration of symptoms in the day.

Role of Fatigue and Drowsiness in RLS

We realized that fatigue or drowsiness could conceivably affect our results. Perhaps leg sensations and PLM were better during the days only because patients were better rested during the days than during the nights. It was therefore possible that the PLM and legs sensations would be worse on the day after sleep deprivation. To look at this we kept the patients up the day after their sleep deprivation night and continued to monitor their leg sensations and PLM. The figure shows that fatigue does make the PLM and leg sensations slightly worse but, again, the shape of the circadian curve is unaltered.

Normal versus Abnormal Circadian Pacemaker in RLS

This data is all suggestive of circadian rythmicity. However, a final question had to be answered: is the circadian rhythm for leg sensations and PLM generated by a circadian pacemaker (suprachiasmatic nucleus of the hypothalamus) that is functioning normally or abnormally?

To answer this question we looked at another circadian rhythm, i.e., the rhythm that is thought to be most closely related to the sleep-wake cycle – body temperature. Our results (not shown in figure) indicate that body temperature in RLS patients has the normal daily rises and falls, being at the lowest point during the night and higher during the day. We also discovered that the PLM and leg sensations are worse at night when body temperature is near its lowest. Therefore, RLS does not seem to be a circadian rhythm abnormality in the same sense as the delayed or advanced, non-24 hour or irregular sleep wake syndromes. Rather, a normal circadian pacemaker is triggering an abnormal response more at certain times of the 24 hour day than at others.

Future Experiments

In the future we plan to repeat these experiments, this time allowing patients to move around in bed as much as they want during the three nights and days. In this way, we can look at the circadian rhythm of motor restlessness. We also plan to use bright artificial sunlight to reset the biological clock to new time zones to see what effect this will have on leg sensations, motor restlessness and PLM. We can predict that we will be able to do this since RLS patients from two countries have independently reported to Dr. Trenkwalder and me that they get their symptoms at the wrong time for the new day immediately after transatlantic flight. However, within a week, the sunlight in the new time zone has reset their circadian biological clocks and, again they are getting their symptoms at night. In addition, we plan to look at melatonin, a natural sleep substance whose production is linked to the circadian pacemaker. Melatonin is made only at night by the pineal gland. What will it do to the circadian rhythm of RLS?

Arthur S. Walters, M.D.
Department of Neurology
Robert Wood Johnson Medical School
New Brunswick, New Jersey and
VA Medical Center, Lyons, New Jersey

Claudia Trenkwalder, M.D.
Neurologische Klinik
Max-Planck Institute for Psychiatry
Munich, Germany

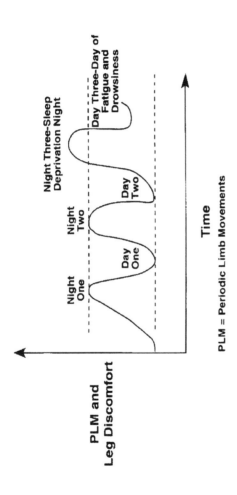

Schematic representation of results of our circadian rhythm study in RLS. The number of periodic leg movements (PLMS) both awake and asleep and leg sensations are plotted versus time. PLMS were recorded for three nights and three days. Leg sensations were rated by the patients on a 1-10 scale for three days and during the night of sleep deprivation. PLMS and leg sensations are worse during the night than during the day and are influenced only slightly by sleep and fatigue.

SECTION IV

Problems that Beset RLS Victims

Chapter One

Sex, Marriage, and RLS with "A Love Letter to My Spouse"

by Virginia N. Wilson

The editor of the *RLS Night Walker* received the question, "Does having sex stop restless legs?" The question was printed in a later issue of the newsletter. Few answers were received, but one from a young man was quite memorable, "Yes! For about eight minutes."

The urge to move may foster strong feelings that a sexual climax might put an end to involuntary leg movements, at least for one night, but that seems to be a false hope. This is not a scientific answer from controlled research but from personal experience, conversations with and letters from various ages and sexes of RLS sufferers. The author has reached the conclusion that the young man was correct in his analysis. The same answer holds true for masturbation which may seem to be the answer to a severe attack, but the truth is, the temporary relief comes from the motion involved rather than sexual gratification.

"When things don't work well in the bedroom, they don't work well in the living room either." William H. Masters' statement certainly relates to the relationship in which one partner is afflicted with RLS. It is possible, even probable, that sex will present problems and that the bedroom may become a battle zone for the couple who must adjust to the unwelcome intruder who shares the connubial bed. This sleep thief has no conscience and uses many alibis like "I'm too tired."

The partner who says "I'm too tired." is not lying. Going without sleep and walking miles during wee hours, then trying to function as a normal person with tasks to perform during the daytime, drains every ounce of energy from the night walker. Going to bed is looked upon as a two-sided Janus head. One face hopes that the bed will wrap its loving arms about the night walker and heavenly sleep will instantly smother even the slightest tickle of an RLS attack, while the other face knows the spouse is looking forward to a romantic sexual romp. The problem does not end when the satisfied partner immediately drops off into a deep, restful sleep; it is but the beginning for the night walker's restless legs to force "I'm too tired" to get up from the comfortable bed to walk, walk, walk – alone – in a shadowy house with night lights marking the familiar path between the rooms. Resentment boils within the patient while murmuring, "It isn't fair."

At last, when the leg sensations diminish, the night walker drops onto the living room sofa to snatch a short nap rather than disturb the bed partner who lies stretched out on the queen-sized bed, peacefully enjoying the last daybreak hours of deep slumber. This becomes a nightly ritual. The wool afghan feels warm. The night walker drifts off into sleep when the sun begins to streak the eastern sky.

Again resentment blossoms with the rude awakening words, "Why are you sleeping out here in the living room? Why do you leave our bed every night? Afraid I'll touch you? If that's the way you feel about me I can sleep in the spare room! I sure don't want to keep you from your bed!" ending with heavy footed steps and the harsh echoes of slammed doors. After that spurt of verbal venom the night walker slowly gathers up the knitted afghan, folds it, carefully places it over the end of the sofa and slowly walks into the kitchen, hoping a cup of coffee will ease the heartache of another failed encounter and dispel the headache that insists playing leap frog in the brain.

This scenario, played all too often, breaks down the love bonds that hold a marriage together. Fear of losing the spouse frightens both parties. The specters of unfaithfulness and disaffection rise. The unseen thief of sleep makes both parties vulnerable unless RLS is recognized as a physical disorder, one that can be treated with proper medication. The couple should learn about this disorder together so that this marriage can last and be rewarded with deep affection. Love partners must learn to share emotions. The female RLS victim must let her partner know the panic she experiences when she is forced, by habit or custom, to accept male dominance while she fights the terrible surge of wanting to get out of the bed and walk. Today's woman should not be afraid to suggest other times or positions that do not make her experience the feeling of being trapped. She should not fear insulting her mate's ego. Love making is love sharing. Bette Davis said in the movie, *The Lonely Life,* "Love is not enough. It must be the foundation, the cornerstone – but not the complete structure."

Learning that there are millions of people all over the world, up to twelve million in the United States alone, who suffer from this syndrome, dispels beliefs that the night walker spouse is fabricating destructive actions that interfere with daily living. With understanding and patience, marriages and relationships can be saved and become full expressions of love.

Proper medication is an important tool in helping marriages work, but it is very important to realize that sometimes medications do not work. Sometimes an RLS victim will have an attack in a restaurant and will have to stand while finishing the meal. The spouse helps by not becoming nervous and making remarks such as, "Sit down. Everybody is looking at us."

Quite often a walk to the rest room will calm the jittery leg muscles, but if that fails it is important to ignore what other people might think. The victim should stand up and flex the legs slightly at the knee. Chances are the diners are busy eating and talking and really don't care what anyone else is doing. (However, one time I did have a lady send me a message with the waitress about how I could rub vinegar on my legs and the cramps would stop. I nodded my thanks to her and received a broad smile in return. I never did try that remedy. Perhaps I should.) Waitresses are usually very sympathetic. They often have leg cramps from being on their feet for so long. If the attack continues, I have put dabs of food on a saucer and eaten while giving a light stomp of the foot now and then, like a horse getting rid of flies. Just thinking of the horse may start a chuckle. A good laugh always helps. As suddenly as the problem appears, the restless discomfort may disappear and dessert may be eaten while sitting at the table. Such an event is not a major catastrophe. Unexpected attacks are annoying, but they need not destroy the social life completely worrying it might happen again. If planning to attend a banquet as a couple, be sure that an exit is close by. Quietly leaving a table will not create a scene that might embarrass your companion. Being thoughtful of each other is the primary rule of living happily with RLS.

Attending a musicale, a movie, a talent show or even a child's graduation ceremony may become another battleground. Be prepared. Whoever buys the tickets or selects seats should think ahead. A seat on the outside aisle avoids two potential hazards: sitting in the middle seat in a ten seat tier while trying desperately to hold quivering legs quiet or stepping over five pairs of feet while murmuring, "Pardon me." The same advice holds true for Sunday morning church services or your child's graduation exercises.

Stand up, go to the rear and enjoy! Remember the show looks the same from the back of the theater and the sermon message is identical in the narthex. Your jumpy legs will disturb no one. Be especially loving to your partner on the way home. That will be thanks enough for having to finish the program sitting next to an empty seat.

A happy marriage is not proof of how compatible the partners are, but proof of how the partners cope with incompatibility. Sex is an important part of any marriage or relationship, but it is only one facet of making a partnership work. Love is deeper than just sharing sex. Actually great obstacles can strengthen a relationship and certainly RLS is an obstacle that is difficult to accommodate for both the victim and the spouse. Sometimes the RLS sufferer feels the strain of trying to carry on a "normal" daily life is almost insurmountable, but with a caring and understanding partner life can go on in an almost normal way. Revealing this physical problem to members of the family, spouse, mother, father, brothers, sisters, children, and especially the in-laws, makes the impossible become possible. Sharing information about RLS with others enriches the patient's life. Helping others understand the mysterious sleep thief is one of the most important duties of every Night Walker.

Try writing a love letter to your spouse. This is the one I have written to my husband Jack:

My darling,

I know that you love me and I also know that sometimes you are angered by my seeming disinterest in your exciting plans for a vacation, ranging from a camping week-end to an African safari.

Even though you know I have the restless legs syndrome, you believe that by taking my prescribed medication I should be able to live as normal a life as you do. After all these years you still *forget that RLS does not completely disappear with medication. It only lessens in intensity, sometimes. Even though I take my pills regularly, medication often fails me. You'd think I'd find something that would give relief that I could **count** on. Not so! I am just as disappointed with the failures as you are, but somehow you seem to forget the agony I suffer as I try to ignore my symptoms to please you. I do want to keep you happy, but I approach each "vacation" with apprehensions. Will I be able to do what you think is fun? I wish I could look forward to each trip as a pleasure, whether it be a jaunt in the car to a camp site in the mountains or jet-journey to a distant city, but I must look upon either of them as something I may have to endure. **Endure**: that is the key word.*

Being able to endure or cope is my definition of a good time now. But sometimes I could liken a vacation to being placed in a medieval torture chamber – stretched on a rack where honey has been poured over my legs to invite ants and rats to gnaw upon my flesh.

We start every vacation late. I simply can't trip off at the crack of dawn especially if I've had my usual restless night. I'm sorry I ask you to stop so many times for me to get out and stretch, only to have to ask you again soon, but you know that I have trouble sitting for any length of time. What you don't know is that I pray a short prayer every time we start out anyplace that this time will be different and I will not have an RLS attack on the way. But my legs have minds of their own. "Move!" They tickle with a feather light touch. I try to ignore them, pretend nothing is happening. Suddenly my legs muscles demand to get out of the car and stretch. I roll my head back, close my eyes and inwardly hum a mantra, "sheama, sheama, sheama," over and over, trying to block out the rising discomfort that is taking over half of my body. I shudder and tighten my leg muscles, tighter, tighter, hoping that you won't notice my twisting and turning.

If you notice, you don't mention it as you drive along the highway and chat happily, "Won't it be great getting away from the house and living close to nature for a week?"

Then I say, "There's a rest station up ahead, let's stop. I need to walk."

"Stop? We've only been gone thirty minutes. We'll never get to the campsite before dark if we stop every thirty minutes along the way." Your voice has a slight edge to it.

I'm sorry, dear, for all the trips I have made miserable for you! And I regret all the times I've had to leave my seat beside you in church or at the theater while I stand in the back, marching in place. Step, step, step. And the times I embarrass you in restaurants while I stand to finish my meal and move my legs as inconspicuously as I can manage. The waitress comes by, looks at me and asks, "Cramps in your legs?" You smile graciously as I nod my reply. Eating out is not always a fun event. Without complaint, you understand when I say "no" to your offer and go to the kitchen to microwave a couple of frozen dinners.

You absolutely abhor my getting up from a banquet table which leaves an empty chair beside you. If I were to stay, the jolting of my body would be worse. I'm glad you understand.

My attention span is shortened when RLS takes over. When we are partners at the bridge table and I am forced to get up and walk between my turns, I often lose the thread of the game and flub my crucial play of the evening. You're a good loser and put your arm around my shoulders to give me a reassuring hug when maybe you really want to throttle me for playing into an obvious trap I missed.

I thank you for helping me with the myriad tasks I once performed easily. Now I am so tired they become mountains for me to climb.

I appreciate your not making a fuss when I leave our bed every night to pace the floor. You know I love the feel of your body next to mine but when the twitching starts I have to get up. I'm thankful that even fire-engine sirens don't disturb your sleep.

Living with an RLS victim requires much love and patience. You give me both or I could never survive. When I sink into a hole of desperation you come to my rescue, not with a 911 call, but with a tender hug and "I know you're having a rough time" smile. I love you for helping me when my legs become like, as Carol Walker says, "motors with no cut-off switches."

How I relish your smile of joy when the RLS releases me and my body quiets. It's like old times again. Together we prepare hot popcorn to eat while we sit on the sofa and laugh at a Benny Hill video. Who cares if I have to stand up and walk every once in a while?

My darling, I love you!

Virginia

Chapter Two

When Panic Sets In: Simple Rules to Follow to Calm Down

by Virginia N. Wilson

Restless Legs attacks take over my life. There is no ignoring the jumping legs and even when they are not jumping much of the time there is a disagreeable sensation – a creepy drawing feeling which makes the skin feel taut. All this and the feeling of lack of control cause nervousness. Unfortunately, while medication sometimes help me get to sleep, the constant weariness and drugs make life miserable, so writes Mary, a 76-year-old woman in Crystal River, Florida, as she states the problem of many.

When the body will not quiet, even after medication, when the household is asleep and the rooms are dark, when the legs insist on pacing or dancing about the floor while the head begs to lie quietly on a pillow and the heart begins to pound – that is the moment when panic strikes.

Panic is a normal reaction to stress. Fatigue is stressful, there is no doubt, and into the stressed brain all the turmoils of living roll and roil about. "Why? Why Me? Why me?" the brain whispers, then shouts, "Why must I walk, walk, walk?" There are about 12 million Americans who may sometime come to experience this pinnacle of stress, called panic. The thought of suicide runs through this turmoil. The RLS patient must not give way to destructive thoughts that bounce around in a sluggish, tired brain.

"Alone in the dark, I came to the conclusion that suicide was my only way out, but as a Christian with a wonderful husband and family I knew I couldn't do it. I became wildly hysterical."

Fran knows all about panic. She has learned to live with it. With proper medication she has less stressful nights, but she doesn't expect to live stress free. She is learning to cope with RLS.

Losing control of any part of the body is frightening and, when the whole body refuses to respond to the need for rest, it is overwhelming. That is a good time to remember the other millions of victims who may be going through the same problem at that very hour. If you had a chance to talk to Jesse in Jersey City who is also pacing the floor and maybe going through a suicidal experience, what would you say to him?

"Hello, Jesse? This is Phil in Philadelphia. I'm a fellow RLS sufferer and I'm having a terrible night. I need to talk to someone. I can't sit down, I can't lie down. I'm frantic. I'm pacing the floor around and around. I've done everything I can think of: I've taken my medicine, I've exercised – ran three miles – took a warm shower, every damn thing I can dream up and I'm still prancing around like an idiot."

And Jesse says, "I know what you mean. I'm doing the same thing. Think I'm going nuts and so does my family."

"You, too? Thought I was the only one in the whole damn world that had RLS so bad."

"Been thinking of suicide all evening. That would end it all. You got a family?"

"Yeah. That's all that keeps me from jumping out a twenty story building – except I can't sit in the car long enough to get to a twenty story building."

"Been thinking about blowing my brains out – guess I'm chicken."

"Might try drowning."

"In a bathtub? Hell, I'm twenty miles from the ocean."

"How about pills. Don't you have some that would do the job? Think that might be relaxing for a while at least."

"Not me. Anything that's supposed to quiet me makes me run. I want to be sure to do the job completely. I'd hate to try and fail."

"Could put a plastic bag over your head!"

"How about you? You got a bag you could use? We could do this thing together right now!"

Maybe twenty to thirty minutes later, after exchanging ideas for the best way to commit suicide, you and Jesse would be laughing at all the crazy ideas. You feel a sense of relaxation wave over you. "Well, Jesse, old Buddy. Thanks to you, I'm beginning to mellow out and I think maybe I can sleep now."

"I was just thinking the same thing, Phil. Anytime you need me, just call. You know, you helped me through a devil of a night, too."

"Well, we both know we didn't imagine all this. It can't be just us, Jesse. It's got to be the weather."

"You know the old saying, everybody talks about the weather and nobody does anything about it! Good night, Phil."

As the long-time editor of the *Night Walker Newsletter* many of the readers know my name and phone number, so it isn't surprising that I get a lot of long-distance calls from frantic people late in the night. We talk and talk about anything and when I hear the caller laugh at something one of us said, I know the panic attack is over. It's a good feeling to hear that laugh. The night walker has risen to the crest of a crisis and slid down a wave to safety. Sometimes it takes thirty minutes, but to the one suffering from panic, it can be the beginning of a lifetime for someone who is so desperately in need of an understanding friend. It is important for both the caller and the listener.

Many times when my own legs will not stay quiet long enough for me to sit even a minute I hear the phone ring and while I am pacing the floor I get strength by telling the caller to take some deep breaths and try to calm down. It's a good "getting to know you time" while the caller pours out all the pain in the brain and in the legs, too. Just talking to a sympathetic listener, one who understands and has experienced this same panic, helps. My own aggravations melt away and become trivial beside the enormous load my caller is carrying because I KNOW my condition is temporary. We both gain and regain the control that had driven us to the edge of panic.

I like to recall the "Golden Rules for Coping with Panic" by Ann Landers that I cut out of the newspaper several years ago. I have revised them to help others through RLS panic attacks.

1. Remember that though the feelings and symptoms you are experiencing are frightening, they are neither dangerous nor life threatening. Take time to take ten deep breaths, as deep as you can make them and hold them as long as you can before exhaling. This will increase the oxygen supply to your brain and your whole body.

2. Know that what you are experiencing is merely an exaggeration of normal reactions to stress. Your heart may beat a bit faster and that is indeed normal – the old "run from danger" adrenal rush.

3. Remember – fighting the feelings that you might explode or trying to wish them away are futile. Recognize the fact that your need to move about is real, physical, and **temporary.** You know it does go away, maybe a bit slower than you'd like, but it **does** go away in time.

4. Remember, there will be an end to your legs misery. You may be one of those who are affected by the change in the weather. This is not considered scientific, but many Night Walkers find their legs

respond negatively to the rise or fall of the barometer. Listen to the weather report. There may be a storm somewhere near you. The rise and fall of the barometric pressure sometimes affects a person suffering from arthritis, rheumatism, headaches, and any number of maladies. You can't do anything about the weather! Don't be a Don Quixote fighting against invincible odds. As an old auntie of mine always reminded me, "There's an end to everything." If the barometer falls, it does rise again!

5. Don't dwell on your fear that this might get worse. Stay in the present and be aware of what is happening to you and think of ways to relieve the pain and insistent need to walk.

6. Count your uneasiness level from zero to ten and watch it go up and down. Notice that it doesn't stay at level ten for more than a few seconds.

7. Change your "what if" thinking. Think of something to do. Work on your computer. Stand up at the kitchen counter and play solitaire. Get at the ironing you've put off for weeks. Any simple, manageable task that you can perform even if you have to jump up and down while you do it. Keeping the brain active seems to help the anxiety wear itself out. One Night Walker writes that she listens to a VCR of Van Cliborn playing the piano, and her RLS leaves.

8. Be aware of the moment when you stop thinking frightening thoughts and peace begins to creep over your body.

9. Wait and let the quiet enfold you. Don't be in a hurry. Think about how good you **will** feel when the anxiety has passed completely.

10. Think of how much better you feel than you did hours ago. Relish that moment of peace when you are in total control. It's time to go back to bed and sleep.

11. (Added) And if all this fails, try soaking in a tub of warm water or loll in a Jacuzzi.

Doctors seldom witness an extreme RLS panic attack in the office so there is small wonder that this disorder is still a mystery. A patient may take a prescription for years and it works most of the time, but, and this is a big word BUT, sometimes it fails completely and the night walker does endure agonies that are indescribable.

There is no way to express what victims endure. Being forced to walk when the legs want to lie or sit quietly and the head begs to watch a TV show or even read a book is a torture that cannot be expressed clearly enough for a mate to understand. No one should expect someone else to completely comprehend this compulsion so the victim should work out leg problems alone. Even a devoted mate tires of RLS complaints because they are often repetitive and hopeless to assist. (Unless a gentle hour long massage is offered to relieve tired muscles.)

The night walkers must work out the best possible medical regimes with a physician's help. If they have more than one ailment, with a specialist for each, they need to take their bottles of assorted prescribed medicines and over-the-counter pills, to the RLS doctor. It is vital to keep records of what times and amounts of medication do the best body regulating, noting on the paper any unusual reactions. Try to take medication on time. Do not wait until a panic attack strikes because waiting until the tickling or cramps begin is TOO late for the medicine to help. It takes twenty to thirty minutes for almost every medication to be assimilated into the body. Thinking ahead is an important part of keeping the body calm. (I must confess that sometimes I'm busy and forget to take my medication until it's too late. Please don't do as I do. Watch it! Don't skip a pill time.)

Also it is vitally important to know RLS medications' time limitations. If a pill is programmed to last two or three hours, it can't be expected to extend its magic all night. (This causes many patients to have miserable experiences when a physician prescribes one 25/100 carbidopa, levodopa at bedtime). The patient may gets some welcome sleep only to wake up in two or three hours. If the doctor doesn't tell the patient about the life span of the medication he prescribes, that it needs to be replenished when its strength is used up, the patient becomes bewildered and cries out, "It failed me. Just like all the rest. It worked for a few hours and then I woke up and couldn't get back to sleep." Ask your pharmacist for the printed sheet that comes with your medication and check the half-life time references.

The pharmacist's sheet may also be able to answer the question, "Why isn't my medication working? Why do I need to have more and more and it still doesn't help?" **Remember more is not always better.** Some insert sheets actually say to try cutting the pill in half if more seems to be needed. Every patient has to work out his or her own best possible individually tailored medical regime and must accept the responsibility of finding the best blend for his/her own body. No doctor can be with a patient 24 hours a day. Remember that what helps one does not always help another. Finding a caring physician to talk this over with is extremely important.

Not only is it important to design and keep a medical chart, the patient must invent ways to cope with family needs. RLS patients must never forget the family needs. Wise patients know that early mornings may be absolute wash-outs, so they don't plan early morning outings. Know limitations and try to live within them. If lovemaking with your mate is impossible at night, when RLS strikes viciously, make plans to be lovey-dovey at a more acceptable hour. Living in any RLS household becomes an exacting balancing act. Think of each day as a performance in the circus with incredible showmanship of coping and hoping for a better tomorrow.

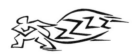

Chapter Three

Worry Over Holding a Job

by Virginia N. Wilson

Personally, I never had to worry about losing my job because of my restless legs. During my high school years I always sought holiday and vacation jobs clerking in retail stores. My restlessness didn't bother me because I was on the go all the time and loved it. Probably made me a good salesperson.

My school days ended at the peak of the 1929-30 depression. I could not go on to college because in those days scholarships meant tuition only. Since my father lost his job, I tried to work to meet living expenses at school, but my health failed. Jobs were nonexistent so I created one, a walking job.

I walked from house to house for a local wholesale bakery. During the week I handed out little wax paper sacks containing two slices of a new vitamin D bread. Saturdays found me in grocery stores with a card table decorated with trays of fancy sandwiches filled with cheese and raisins or cheese and onions. Evenings I gave lectures and refreshments at school P.T. A. meetings and union halls where I was introduced as the sales manager of the firm. I earned two dollars a day and was glad to get that. Years later the owner who had hired me told me that when I came in that morning he was cutting the payroll to keep from having to close his bakery and I had convinced him I could make money for him. That company is still in operation today, although with new owners, so walking and restlessness gave me a job and saved a business!

After several years with the bakery came the years of raising a family. This was the time when I began to notice my inability to sleep and when I did sleep I always seemed to be on the edge of waking up. When our first child, Marilyn, was less than one year old she developed a severe case of croup, a well known malady of Illinois snowbound winters. To relieve her coughing I rigged up a "steamer" by placing a small electric plate beside her bed to keep steaming menthol vapors rolling into her sheet-shrouded crib. Exhausted, I lay down upon our bed, only feet away from the crib and dropped off to sleep. A sudden flare of flames engulfed the crib. Somehow the sheet fell onto the electric burner and caught fire. I rushed to pull the flaming sheet to the floor, covered it with a throw rug, and in that terrible moment I realized how stupid I had been. In my groggy condition I had foolishly almost burned my child and the house. I thought this incident could be the "cause" of my insomnia. From then on I blamed my problem on the physical and mental demands of being a mother.

Years later my husband and I bought a combination floral and gift shop, and hobby shop. He managed the hobbies and did all the accounting work for both stores while I wore many hats as floral manager, buyer, salesperson, designer, lecturer, demonstrator, and general do-what-ever-needs-to-be-done person. All the while I was plagued with insomnia. I was chronically tired. My husband often fussed because he would find me on the davenport almost every morning. I had long blamed my inability to sleep on the children, but now they were grown and gone. So I changed the blame to my work, believing that I was too tired to rest. Of course that was backwards thinking, but to the RLS victim it is logical backwards reasoning. After all, you have to blame SOMETHING! There simply HAS to be a reason!

I could hardly wait to sell our stores so that I would be able to rest. I was convinced that my life would change – that I could sleep like a normal person – with the removal of the pressures of running the business, the watching over past due accounts, the assuaging of customers and help all day, every day, every week, every month, year in and year out. I had had it! My husband always looked forward to remaining a hobby shop entrepreneur growing old and maybe even senile on the job but I couldn't take it any more. I was so tired I could barely drag myself to work. If I had been an employee, I would have been scolded or even fired. But of course, no one ever questioned the store owner's right to be weary.

Retirement didn't help. Even in a new house in a new Florida environment the lack of sleep still dogged me. I was worse at leisure than I had been at work. I still walked the floor night in and night out. Little did I realize then that millions of others were struggling with this same problem. I questioned my sanity until I learned that I suffered from RLS.

In 1990, after I began corresponding with other RLS patients, I realized what devastating results come from ignorance. These letters from RLS victims make us realize that many men and women, all ages and skills, are dealing with a serious disability creating great mental hurdles for them every day. Probably one of the most important hurdles is the worrying over being unable to continue working:

Last night I didn't sleep all night because both legs bothered me. That is one of many nights I haven't slept all night. I really feel depressed because the bad news is I have been making so many mistakes on my job I'm going to get fired and I do need the money. It is hard to concentrate when you feel like you want to go to sleep. I haven't told them my problem, but it sounds like they are eager to get rid of me.

M. F., Olympia, Washington

It [RLS] has ruined my life. I was a police officer in Ohio and could not ride with anyone because of my legs. If I drove it wasn't so bad. I was injured on the job and had to have back surgery and lost my job. After the surgery they couldn't understand in the hospital why I couldn't sleep because of my legs. That was back in 1978. I was forced to retire. After I retired they tried so many drugs it changed me so much it cost me my twenty-eight-year-marriage. Even my dog can't sleep with me. I get a total of three to four hours of sleep but not over two hours at one time. I have gotten up and in the dark just started taking drugs trying to overdose. I have been on medication so long my body has adjusted to it. I take anywhere from five to ten pills (pain medication) at bedtime and they don't help, but I'm stuck on them and can't break free. They just dull the brain for a few hours. Every day I think I can't go on with no rest, but I manage like other people. I have been to sleep clinics with no help! My doctor said I have the worst case she has every seen. At age fifty-two I'll probably never see any relief in my life but maybe someday there will be a cure.

D. M., Port Charlotte, Florida

I am no longer able to work in an office as I once did, because I cannot sit at a desk for very long. I really can't decide which is worse: not being able to sleep at night, or not being able to sit or rest during the day. There are days when the anxiety is almost too much to bear.

L. I., Aston, Pennsylvania

I am having a very difficult time, ten years now, with this syndrome. My mother had it, my son has it, and my daughter, but not as bad as me. I have had it every night as soon as I go to bed and it lasts until five or six or seven in the morning. It's in my hips and legs and causes me pain from all the thrashing around. I have no energy during the day and want to sleep all day. My life has totally changed. I was a legal secretary for thirty-two years and now I can hardly get my dishes done. This past year I have been in a depression over it.

PS. I am now 62 years old and would like to have the energy to enjoy my life and my grandchildren.

E. T., Pointe Claire, Quebec

Since the age of six, for the past thirty-two years I have been seeking help from one doctor to another. After all these years and fifty plus physicians that I have seen I finally have been diagnosed with RLS. I've tried every medication possible and am now on $150-200 per month for medicine.

I am having terrible difficulties dealing with this disease because it has rendered me disabled and I cannot meet my potential in life.

J. H., Navarre, Florida

I was a long distance truck driver for over twenty years. I've been unable to work since December 1990. In May 1990 I went to . . . Sleep Disorder Center and was told I had a severe sleep disorder due mainly to periodic leg movements.

I'm fifty-four years old. For the last four years my weight has stayed at 240 to 250. I gained thirty to forty pounds between 1988 and 1990 eating crunchy foods to stay awake while driving. I was also eating just before I went to bed hoping it would help me sleep. Many nights it takes a half hour or more to go to sleep. An hour or so later I'm awake. It takes thirty minutes or more to go back to sleep then. A half hour or so later I'm awake again, then the sleep time starts decreasing to twenty, fifteen, or ten minutes. During the time I say I'm sleeping, many times I wake up long enough to change position or just lie awake.

Even though I haven't worked since 1990 my sleep problem hasn't changed. I have a lot of medical problems (which I feel are the result of my sleep problem) but I haven't given up. I hope that someday I might get some help for my problems.

E. S., Boswell, Indiana

It is obvious that all ages and both sexes are vulnerable to the fear of losing jobs. It is time for all of us to consider the high cost of not knowing that RLS is a physical disorder that can be treated with medication. For many, the days are endless because there is no sleep at night to renew the body. Right now we do not have a cure, but with proper medication, and an understanding physician to work with, there is hope that the coming days will be better.

RLS can have a good side. The walking need and the restlessness are often channeled positively in the young. No doubt there are many successful men and women out there who are successful because they have so much energy and can't spend hours sitting or lying in bed.

Most of us are able to cope with this disability when we have a proper diagnosis. It is our privilege and responsibility to help others learn to cope in their daily lives. We need to teach families how to be supportive. We must help others understand the torture of losing control of the body, the embarrassment of having to get up and leave a meeting or the inability to sit while eating.

We must educate our physicians so that we will eliminate all the useless and expensive treatments that most of us have undergone for years, and strive to have RLS taught in medical schools. We can write letters to Washington to seek help for sleep research. No matter how old or infirm we are there is a new profession to explore. EACH ONE TEACH ONE! Spread the word. We must stop this loss of jobs because of the lack of sleep.

Chapter Four

Alcohol and RLS: Is RLS Caused by Alcoholism or Vice Versa?

by Virginia N. Wilson

Luke eased into the chair beside the desk where the white-coated doctor sat and said, "Doc, do you know what the two luckiest days in my life were?"

"No," the doctor said as he turned the pages of Luke's records the nurse had placed on his desk.

"The day I wrecked my truck and got a ticket for DUI, and the day that sawbones doctor called *you* in on my case."

The doctor nodded. "I'd say that is an odd combination of the definition of good days, but I do thank you."

"That night I had my first good sleep in years without drinking God-knows-how-much beer before I could go to bed. You were the first doctor who ever listened! And you were the first who got the picture when I told you my legs were so jumpy and crawly I could never get to sleep. Man, Doc! It's been two whole years since my last drink."

"Yours is not a rare situation, Luke. There are recovering alcoholics like you who are frantic for sleep and they think the beer or wine relaxes them enough to sleep – but it really doesn't do that at all. After a while the nervous system rebels and sleep is more fragmented than ever."

"But I'm telling you, Doc, when you get those twitching legs going you don't know what to do. My poor wife has rubbed my legs until her arms gave out. And there's no way to count how many damned times I've sat in tubs of hot water."

The doctor laughed. "You're right. From the stories I have heard, I believe that RLS people are among the cleanest in the world. That seems to be the general panacea when all else fails."

"You won't believe this, Doc. I've had doctors laugh when I talked about my legs. Some went so far as to wink and make crude remarks about what I needed. And nobody, I mean nobody, listened to me until you did. I'm telling you, if it hadn't been for my wife and knowing I had kids to raise I would have jumped off the top of a tall building – many times."

"Unfortunately, Luke, not much is known about this syndrome. Even though it's been around for many years it hasn't been taken seriously – say like heart attacks or strokes, cancer, and diabetes. But what the medical world doesn't seem to understand is that RLS kills, too. Lack of sleep drains the body of its energy. Perception is gone. Accidents happen. People are killed."

"Just knowing I have a disorder with a name helps. I figured I was plumb nuts – the only one in the world who walked most of the night – who dreaded to see the evenings come. When I found out there were a lot of us out there, it sure made a difference. Who would believe that moving, crazy legs could keep you from sleeping? I always thought it was the other way around. I couldn't sleep, so my legs went crazy."

"Well now, I think we're on the right track with you and your medication. We may have to switch to something else one of these days because people sometimes build up tolerances. But we'll work together and find another one for you if we have to. I'm delighted to know that you've successfully passed two years of —"

"Yea, no boozin'. I had enough of trying to get numb to get to sleep. Sure is great not to have a headache and a fuzzy mouth every morning, to say nothing about how thankful my wife is. Funny, but I really never even liked the damned stuff – it just meant getting enough sleep so I could go to work the next day."

...

The chapter on alternative treatments states very positively that the RLSF Medical Advisory Board does not recommend alcohol for sleep disorders since scientific studies have shown that while it may improve sleep for the first half of the night, it disrupts sleep during the second half of the night.

However, it seems that some sleep-deprived victims use alcohol to lull themselves into stupor-slumber in lieu of restful-slumber. Letters written by patients lead me to believe that chronic alcoholism may be a **complication** of RLS. I was delighted to find my theory supported by Dr. Melissa Stoller (Stoller, 1994) in her scholarly report "Economic Effects of Insomnia." She starts the section of her paper entitled, "Insomnia and Alcoholism" with the statement:

"Insomnia may be a causal factor in the development of alcohol abuse and thus contribute to alcohol-related morbidity and mortality. It has been long recognized that there is a significant association between alcohol use and insomnia. The rate of alcoholism among insomniacs is twice that of good sleepers."

Seeming to back up her statement are parts of letters that made me realize how many people try to slay one dragon only to discover a bigger one over the hill.

I used large quantities of alcohol with the excuse that it helped my RLS.

I began drinking alcohol before I went to bed.

During my teens it [RLS] came back. By that time I was using alcohol and drugs.

My grandfather was an alcoholic and he would sit up nights and bang his feet on the floor.

It takes about 12 cans of beer for my son to get to sleep.

One woman from Florida described the starting of her own alcohol abuse:

I have what I call the tickles during the day, but not at all as severe as bedtime. I have gone for days without a decent night's sleep and would come home from work and fix a few cocktails of scotch and water while preparing dinner, drink through dinner, and drink after dinner until I could just lie in bed and pass out. The problem was a lot worse under those conditions and my poor husband went through hell, but the alcohol sedated me enough to sleep through the problem. I normally woke up feeling like I had jogged a twenty mile marathon – and of course, the terrible effects of alcohol. But the satisfaction of getting five to six hours of sleep seemed to make it worth it.

Dr. Stoller states that 60% of alcohol abusers use alcohol to self-treat the inability to go to sleep and stay asleep. Of that 60%, 15.7% indicated that alcohol abuse developed **after** a sleeping disorder, so with this data perhaps it is reasonable to estimate that 9% to 10% of alcohol abuse is the consequence of sleep deprivation.

A number of studies indicate that alcohol abuse may be one of the single most costly health problems in America. The U.S. Department of Health and Human Services places the cost of alcohol abuse between $85 billion and $115 billion per year which includes reduced productivity and increased unemployment of abusers, accident expenses, the untimely deaths, plus the medical care of the chronically ill – to say nothing of the costs of dysfunctional families.

Assuming that the lack of sleep causes 10% of those costly billions, it seems that treatment of sleep deprivation should be addressed aggressively to solve part of this major problem in America. The fact that many RLS undiagnosed and unmedicated victims become alcohol abusers, who add financial and emotional burdens to our families and communities, should be another important reason why we must make the medical world and general public aware of the truth that RLS is a serious physical and treatable disorder.

Chapter Five

Are You a Danger to Yourself and to Others?

By Virginia N. Wilson

One night a man called and asked, "Can you help me? I'm having a very bad RLS attack."

"I'll try," I replied and talked to him in my usual manner, trying to calm his fears and anxiety. His voice sounded young but tired, certainly without vigor or enthusiasm. In my routine questioning to help him to relax and to establish a warm friendly rapport, I asked, "What do you do for a living?"

"I'm an airline pilot. I've got to get some sleep so I can work tomorrow."

His answer caught me off guard, all but completely floored me. Here was a young man, desperately needing sleep, possibly not able to function with the mental agility needed in case of an emergency in the air, who was going to pilot a plane (full of unsuspecting passengers). Actually my hair felt like it was standing on end in fright. What if he were the one who would be piloting my plane on my next air journey?

I answered quickly, "Some people experience mysterious remissions, but I suggest that you think about another line of work. RLS does not get better. It tends to increase with age. Medication is helpful, but not always the giver of the gift of sleep. However, your age is working for you and since you are young, maybe the cause will be found and then a cure – before your productive years are over. For the present time my advice to you is to find the very best doctor you can. Ask him if he knows anything about RLS. If he says, "Yes," stay with him and enter into a partnership of trial and error medicating because that is necessary to survive in an RLS world."

When we see the flight crew walking briskly toward the cockpit of the plane we will be entering soon we see young men or women in well-tailored uniforms and assume they are alert, rested, full of vigor and ready for any action that they might be called upon to perform. We must be aware that this may not true. My fears were alerted again when this letter came in.

What worries me is that I am 31. I don't have RLS all the time, but I do have it in my right leg now and then. I understand RLS gets worse with age and it may some day interfere with my profession. I am an airline pilot.

D. S., Tampa, Florida

What else could I write but the truth as I know it?

Yes, as you age you probably will have added RLS symptoms more frequently. I certainly wouldn't count on it getting less as the years go by.

RLS is one of the many disorders that rob victims of rest. Since it is estimated 2% to 5% of our population suffers from RLS, some of those piloting planes may be victims too. It's rather scary to think of the number of times we trust our lives to those who are not rested. When you ride in a taxi, do you ever wonder if that person driving the cab had walked all night instead of sleeping? And don't we face the same danger every time we go out onto the highway? As you drive along the freeway or even a city street, do you ever wonder about how much sleep that driver behind the steering wheel in that van, car, or a semi-rig coming toward you, had the night before? Our highways are killing fields, often because the drivers are sleep deprived.

I experienced driving while sleep-deprived years ago. We were taking our station wagon loaded with our Illinois household knickknacks to our new Florida home. Just past Louisville, Kentucky, my husband Jack said he was very tired. I volunteered to drive. I knew I hadn't slept the night before but that was normal for me. I had learned to ignore tiredness. I zipped along at 65 miles an hour, listening to the radio while Jack napped peacefully. Suddenly I jolted and woke up, realizing I had dropped off to sleep momentarily. The car was weaving from one side of the four-lane to the other at five miles an hour. A quick glance in my rear view mirror revealed lines of cars creeping along behind me. My adrenaline flowed full force. I stepped on the gas, got out of everybody's way and pulled off the road as quickly as I could. Unaware of our near tragedy Jack woke up. When I told him what had happened, needless to say, he drove all the rest of the way to Florida. I never did offer my long distance driving services again. This was many years before I knew about RLS. Now we all know that sleep deprivation is a major cause of accidents on our highways.

Riding in a car seems to be one of the universal difficulties encountered by RLS victims.

My husband has suffered with this problem [RLS] since he was about sixteen years old and he is now fifty-eight years old. He gets very grouchy and grumpy over driving in the evening. If I drive he can't stand it in the front seat. I have to stop so he can sit in the rear seat and put his legs up on the seat with a rolled up blanket under his knees or lower legs. Sometimes this doesn't work. If he drives, he wants to push the gas pedal through the floorboard of the car.

J. B., Hamburg, Pennsylvania

The sudden loss of control may be the cause of an accident. It is disconcerting to have a sudden shaking spell come over the legs. The desire to press the foot down is great and should be guarded against. Whenever I am driving and come to a red stop light I shift to "park" (even though I have an automatic gear shift) because I fear an unexpected jerk that sometimes comes so rapidly there is no time to think "stop." I certainly don't want to jump suddenly into oncoming traffic. The sound of metal crunching is not music to my ears. If by chance I do have a shaking period come over me, I stop driving and walk around; or if there is a gas station or cafe, I purchase a cup of coffee. (It is an odd phenomenon that many RLS victims can get sudden relief from caffeine. It may be short lived but worth it if your legs insist on running when you can't.) I feel those few minutes spent are not wasted. Also I always have a half-tablet of medication in my purse to get me back to a quietness. I feel that any RLS victim should not ignore these moments of control loss. It only takes a split second to crash into the back of another car and it takes hours to fill out the police and insurance forms, let alone endure the pain of a "whip lash neck." This is another example of the old adage, "A stitch in time saves nine."

In addition to the serious dangers of driving while sleep deprived other problems are often overlooked; for instance, the health caregiver to whom we trust our lives and our family's lives. A lady in Pennsylvania said, "I'm not looking forward to sleepless nights and days of exhaustion. I am a working mother with a husband and two children. I'm in a job where I need to be alert and aware of\ dangerous situations. Lives can depend on how I perform. If I am exhausted from a lack of proper rest, my job performance will certainly suffer and patients that are in my care could be at risk."

I wish I could include the entire letter written by a desperate man because it makes so many points that are relevant to the RLS victim. It is very long, and somewhat rambling and full of medicine references which would not be appropriate to include; however, I want to put a spotlight on the dangers of having RLS and not knowing it. This man entitled his letter "RLS, a Life of Hell" and it truly was one until quite by accident he came across the medication which saved his sanity by taking him from no nightly rest to a five or six hour sleep with which many of us live.

I am now sure my mother had RLS before she died. I couldn't understand why she spent nights beating her legs with her fists and not sleeping. Both my sisters have it as well as I. We knew something was wrong but we referred to it as the "fidgets." We thought it was something some nut in the family tree had passed to us. Much like a curse.

As a medical supervisor of a hospital laboratory and a purchasing agent, I received all kinds of samples of drugs. I found one ___ at bedtime would let me sleep. I used it for several years. Once I had not slept for days and was working almost every night on emergency work such as X-rays of wrecks or getting blood for bleeding patients, so I took a ___ . It did not work so the next night I took two. I was awakened by what I thought was a bright light and pain. I had walked into the edge of a half open door, and hit my head between the eyes. I tried ___ and it put me to sleep but I found that I might get up and walk around or get into the car and drive.

By 1975 I was working for two hospitals as laboratory supervisor in an attempt to cover both for approval by the state. I was working sixteen hours a day and sleeping about two. The problems began to control me then.

K. H., Newport, Tennessee

The rest of the letter goes on to tell of the number of cars he wrecked by falling asleep at the wheel. His life, still without rest, continued to get worse until finally his body developed a series of physical problems. Convinced that he had an incurable mental problem he tried to buy a gun to kill himself but backed off when he had to sign papers at the sheriff's office. In desperation he planned to drive off the end of a bridge into a lake 100 feet below. But he didn't. Later when he visited his sister in a hospital she was given medication to quiet her "jumping legs" and he was amazed when her legs quieted. He asked his own doctor to prescribe the same medicine for his legs. For the first time in years he slept. Later he read a magazine article which described RLS so clearly he knew that he had been suffering from this disorder all his life.

He understands that he isn't cured but he is out of the hell he endured for over twenty years. He's learned that he is not a mental case and he's able to cope with this physical, treatable disorder. The moral of this tale is that had this man been properly diagnosed and treated all those destructive years, his life could have been more satisfying, but as the old saying goes, "Better late than never." I love happy endings!

To be fair to our physicians, the present curricula of medical colleges do not give importance to the causes, nor the serious consequences of sleep deprivation. Is there any wonder that we have so many reports of poor care in the hospital emergency rooms? Doctors and nurses, whom we trust with our own lives, often work long hours and if they have some undiagnosed sleep disorder, which does not allow them to rest properly, the problems of giving care and the danger of receiving care are magnified.

The Washington Post, April 18, 1995, p. A16, reported a suit being filed against a Denver anesthesiologist for going to sleep during a routine ear operation and his child patient died. The prosecutor offered evidence that this same doctor had fallen asleep during six other operations. The doctor is charged with reckless manslaughter. Perhaps the man suffers from a sleep disorder. Isn't it possible that doctors suffer from sleep deprivation in the same ratio as our general populaltion?

Business and professional people alike suffer and wrestle with situations unbecoming to their offices. Nervous "fidgets" come upon RLS victims without warning and without good reason.

As I've grown older, the condition [RLS] has grown much worse. My 83-year-old mother still calls me "Miss St. Vitus" and tells me I could stop it if I wanted to. But I can't and I'm a professional business woman, married with five grown children. Only if you have this problem can you understand the embarrassment of seeing other professionals eye you with uncertainty as they question the advisability of taking advice from someone who sits, constantly shaking her legs.

V. B., Sebring, Florida

I worry whenever I read about a political leader or the head of some large organization who brags that three hours of sleep is enough. We know that is not true. We also know that many of us have existed on two or three hours of sleep at night, off and on, for years. But now the medical world has pronounced that the body cannot go on indefinitely without being recharged by regular, restful sleep. Sleep, once lost, cannot be recovered nor lost rest time made up.

Lack of sleep may trigger depression, and suicide is one of its most dangerous side effects. Letters and messages of despair come to me quite often attesting to that danger, like one from a North Carolina woman whose husband is "so bad [with RLS] some times I fear it could lead to suicide." I get more letters like this than I would wish:

This condition [RLS] has been in our family for many years with no relief for the sufferers. My mother is now ninety-four and is a resident of a nursing home and is much misunderstood because she insists on getting up and walking or thumping her feet on the floor in order to make "her legs lie still." When she tells doctors of this problem they don't even answer her, let alone try and treat her. Her older brother years ago committed suicide because he could no longer tolerate it.

J. H., Carlyle Pennsylvania

We are all aware that RLS is dangerous to our health. This quote rather sums up how many think about this disorder:

Getting two to four hours of sleep at a time, other than that I'm not coping with this stuff at all well. If I had my druthers I would put an end to the "Not Life" I have. There is no pleasure in this existence.

M. M., Yakima, Washington

What is the price the nation pays for the lack of sleep affecting up to 40% of our population? The direct and indirect costs place a large economic burden upon our whole society. A conservative estimate of the total annual cost of insomnia was calculated at $92.5 to $107.5 billion. (Stoller, 1994) These figures include the cost of medical treatment, reduced productivity, absenteeism, alcohol consumption, and depression, as well as death and loss of family income, as sleep loss is a significant cause of accidents on the roads and in the work place.

The purpose of this chapter is to help RLS victims realize that there are grave dangers out there in everyday life and learn how to cope with them. We must all be aware that we are a part of this dangerous world and we are responsible for ourselves and others. We are not alone. There are millions of us who find life very rewarding. We learn to accept and to cope with the problems that this disorder can cause. They are not insurmountable. Throwing up our hands in despair will never solve any problem. We must become an army of the "sleep deprived" fighting for recognition in the medical world. We know the dangers of being ignored. Let information and understanding free us from those dangers.

Note: Details of references in text can be found in Appendix 3, Publications Relating to RLS.

SECTION V

Learning to Cope with RLS

Chapter One

Experiences of Living with a Rare Disorder

Mark Flapan, Ph.D.
(Part two of a three-part series)

Reprinted by permission of the author and the National Organization for Rare Disorders, Inc.

Dr. Mark Flapan has scleroderma and is founder of the Scleroderma Federation of the Tri-State Area. He is a psychologist with a special interest in the emotional effects of chronic illness both on the ill person and on family members

In a previous issue of *Orphan Disease Update*, I wrote about self-pity and self-blame, and about guilt and shame as feelings you don't have to live with. In this issue I'll write about the feeling of hurt which you don't have to suffer as much from either.

With a chronic illness you are more vulnerable to hurt feelings than you would otherwise be. Because of all that goes on inside you, both physically and emotionally, you have a greater need for consideration and signs of concern and caring than you would if you were well and healthy. So when family members and friends don't respond to you in these "understanding" ways, your feelings are hurt.

It may seem that your feelings are hurt by what someone says or does – and that's all there is to it. But that's not all there is to it, not by a long shot. Your feelings are hurt, not by what the other person says or does, but by the meanings you give to what the other person says or does. Different meanings – different feelings.

Your feelings are hurt when a family member or friend says or does something which you take to mean, he's not interested in how you feel, he's not concerned about you, or he doesn't care. The meanings you give come from your understanding of the thoughts and feelings expressed in what the other person says or does – which may or may not be what the other person actually thinks and feels.

A fuller and more accurate understanding of how family members and friends are affected by your illness and what they actually think and feel may alleviate some of your hurt feelings.

Your marital partner

If you're married, it's the reactions of your partner that affect you most. Similarly, it's your partner who is the most affected by your illness. When you consider the effect of your illness on your partner, it should be pointed out that there tends to be a difference between the way wives react and relate to an ill husband and the way husbands react and relate to an ill wife. Women, by and large, are more prepared to accommodate and care for an ill partner than are men.

Beginning with doll play, girls traditionally are raised to take care of children and later as wives are expected to administer to the physical and emotional needs of their husbands – sick or well. Not only that, being an understanding and caregiving person is a more important part of a woman's identity than it is of a man's. Therefore, accommodating the emotional and physical needs of an ill husband is not only more acceptable to women than men, but is more likely to be taken as more of the same.

The unfortunate consequence of this difference, to the extent that it is present, is that more women than men are hurt by their partner's way of relating to their illness. The comments that follow, therefore, are addressed primarily to chronically ill wives but may pertain to ill husbands as well.

Your husband is likely to have complicated feelings related to your illness. He may, for example, be worried about you and afraid you're going to die. And to lessen his fears and yours too, for that matter, he may play down your illness or deny it altogether. He may feel helpless and bewildered about what to do for you and feel inadequate as a caregiver. And if he has never been seriously ill himself, he may be baffled by your reactions to your illness. Even if he has experienced an illness himself, men, by and large, tend to react to and cope differently with physical ailments than do women.

But regardless of his ability to understand what your illness is like for you, he doesn't want to say anything that might hurt or upset you. He's therefore likely to keep his feelings to himself. Or he may be the kind of person who keeps his feelings to himself in any case. Be that as it may, you may experience him as distant and withdrawn rather than as concerned and caring.

To complicate matters more, he's also concerned about himself, which he's even less likely to talk about. While he's saddened by what has happened to you and your life, he's also saddened by the changes in his life as well. After all, you're not as available to him physically or emotionally as you used to be and, more likely than not, he feels deprived and resentful. But what can he say? He knows it's all because of your illness, which neither you nor he, nor anyone else can do anything about.

What may be especially hurtful, if it happens to be the case, is your husband's diminished sexual interest in you. Whether you're interested in sex or not, you want him to find you physically attractive. With a chronic illness, it's hard enough to feel desirable as a wife but it's much harder if your husband loses sexual interest in you.

I'd like to point out, however, that if your husband is worried and depressed by your illness, his sexual needs may also be depressed, and even when he is sexually interested, he may conceal his desire out of concern for you. After all, he knows that your fatigue, your discomforts and your pain may be uppermost on your mind. But if you're unaware that his sexual avoidance may be related to his consideration for you, you'll feel unnecessarily rejected, hurt, and resentful.

In some instances, of course, the effects of a chronic disease do, in fact, diminish a husband's sexual attraction to his wife. When this occurs, he also experiences a sexual loss and wishes it were otherwise. However, this doesn't necessarily mean he loves you any less.

Ironically, if your husband approaches you with some frequency, you may also feel hurt and resentful. You may feel he's not sufficiently sensitive to your physical condition and is primarily interested in satisfying his own needs. In this area it may be that he can't do anything right.

All in all, given what goes on inside him – and much more goes on inside him than what I've mentioned – he may not always respond to you with the sympathetic understanding you need. Unfortunately, when you were given the diagnosis of the disease, he wasn't simultaneously given the emotional wherewithal to deal with it. However, the more fully you understand your husbands's thoughts and feelings related to your illness, the less likely you'll be hurt by misconstruing the meaning of what he says or does.

In addition to trying to understand your partner's thoughts and feelings related to your illness, it's important for you to help him understand yours – not by accusing him of being insensitive and inconsiderate but by being as open as you can about how your illness affects you emotionally. Mutual understanding in a marital relationship is difficult enough, but the addition of a chronic illness requires all the understanding that both the ill and the well partner can come by.

Unfortunately, in some instances, hurt feelings don't come from a lack of understanding but from the well partner's inability to feel the compassion and concern that the ill partner requires. Even before your illness, your partner may not have been particularly thoughtful or considerate, but it didn't matter to you as much then as it does now. Or maybe he's changed since your illness and no longer has the feelings for you he once had. This, of course, is the most hurtful of all.

If this happens to be the case, marital counseling may be helpful if your husband is willing. But whether he is or not, you may have to reconcile yourself to the realization that he doesn't have the feelings required to give you the emotional support you need. In that case you may feel trapped with an illness in an unhappy marriage. But you wouldn't dare leave because you can't imagine who would want you in your condition.

However, your husband doesn't have to be your only source of understanding and support. You may be able to get the understanding and support you need from friends or other family members or from an emotional support group for people with your disease. You need to develop your own inner resources for coping with your illness and thus become less dependent on emotional support from others.

Your children

The way your adolescent and grown children relate to you since your illness may also hurt your feelings. They may show little interest in how you feel and may even have distanced themselves from you. If this is so, keep in mind that at their stage of development, they're still likely to be self-involved. Adolescents are troubled with problems of growing up, and grown children are involved in establishing a long-term relationship. If they're married and have children, they may be troubled with marital or child-rearing problems of their own. The last thing in the world they need is a sick parent to be concerned about.

As a parent, you're not supposed to be sick. You're supposed to be there for them; they're not supposed to be there for you. It's not only your illness that your children may not be able to accept, but the thought of your dying from your disease is too upsetting and frightening for them to even think about.

Grown children, no matter how old, expect their parents to be here forever. While they may think of themselves as independent adults, in their unacknowledged fantasies, you're still their ultimate protector. Your illness threatens all this.

This doesn't mean you might not be able to clarify some areas of misunderstanding by trying to find out specifically how your illness affects them and by telling them how your illness affects you, both physically and emotionally. They may have difficulty being open with you as you may have difficulty being open with them, but openness leads to openness, and it's your first move, like it or not.

Your friends and relatives

With a chronic illness it's inevitable you'll feel more hurt and alienated from friends and relatives than you would otherwise be. It's important to keep in mind, however, that there is no way a person without a chronic disease can understand what it's like to live with one. But why should they understand, they don't have a physical ailment – you do. It's difficult for anyone to understand what he's never experienced. Even with the best of intentions, friends and relatives are going to say and do things that hurt your feelings.

For example, they may ask how you feel when you don't want to be reminded of your illness, or they may not ask how you feel when you want some sign of concern. They may not comfort you when you need it, or may be over solicitous when you're feeling fine. They may not listen to you when you need to talk or listen only impatiently when they do.

If you are visibly affected by your illness, they may pity you – which is demeaning. Worse yet, they may physically distance themselves from you, as if you were contagious. On the other hand, if your illness doesn't show, they may act as if you're not sick at all and expect you to be the same as you always were.

Whether your illness shows or not, our friends and relatives may not understand why you have to break appointments at the last minute. They don't understand "good days and bad days." And since they don't understand they may not invite you to some activity they think you're not up to. But whether you're up to it or not, you want to be invited anyway, and your feelings are hurt when you're not.

As with your husband and children, you may not fully understand how your illness affects your friends and relatives, and you may, at times, misconstrue the meaning of what they say and do. Only by openly talking with them about how their behavior affects you, and by learning how your illness affects them, can you find out what's really going on. To be realistic, however, don't expect complete understanding from friends and relatives, otherwise you'll continue to feel disappointed and hurt.

But what's most hurtful of all is the rejection of friends you don't hear from anymore. How could they abandon you when now, more than ever, you need friends who care? Unfortunately, you may have no choice but to grieve the loss of friends brought on by your illness and try to make new friends – as difficult as it may be with your illness.

You're single

If you're single and trying to meet people and establish a relationship, you're especially vulnerable to hurt feelings. If your illness shows, your feelings are hurt when someone you're interested in turns away from you. If your illness doesn't show, you have the problem of when and what to say about your condition. And when you do decide to tell a person you're going with about your illness, and he loses interest in you – you're not only hurt but devastated.

This rejection is especially hurtful because it confirms your feeling of being undesirable. To relieve your hurt feelings, you need to develop a sense of worth <u>as a person with an illness</u>.

Your parents

In some cases your parents may also be a source of hurt feelings. When you were sick as a child, one or both of your parents may have been caring and comforting. Now that you're ill as an adult, your parents may not be there for you as they once were.

Your parents, in their present stage of life, are likely to be worried about matters that didn't concern them when you and they were younger. They may be concerned about their own physical ailments and uneasy about how much time they have left. Or if it's not their own health and life they're primarily concerned about, they may be worried about the health and aging of their partner. This frightens them with the prospect of living the rest of their life alone.

Your parents are not likely to tell you, their "child," about these and other fears related to aging. This doesn't mean you can't initiate such a conversation. This would not only enable you to understand them better but, in all likelihood, would bring you closer together. Here, as in your other relationships, the more completely you understand what your parents are going through, the less likely you'll feel hurt by their self-involvement and their seeming indifference to your illness. In fact, you may even discover that their feelings are hurt by your not taking greater interest in the ailments.

The situation is different, however, if your parents were never particularly understanding or caring. Their lack of present concern is likely to evoke old hurt feelings. It's also likely to evoke feelings of being unworthy now, as it did when you were a child. If that's the case, you have more to understand about yourself and your relationship with your parents over the years. Keep in mind, however, it's unlikely you'll be able to get from them now what you didn't get from them before. But you don't have to blame yourself for it.

When all is said and done

It's your responsibility to establish and maintain the best relationships you can in spite of your illness. This includes learning as much as you can about how your illness affects others emotionally and helping them understand how your illness affects you emotionally as well as physically. You may even learn, in the process, that you're putting people off by the way you're acting. If that's the case, you may have to change some of your ways if you're going to get the understanding and consideration you want.

But even if you change your ways and increase your and other's understanding of the emotional effects of your illness, you're still not likely to get all the support you want.

It's therefore important to strengthen your inner resources for coping with your illness. By strengthening your own inner resources, you will have less need for emotional support from others and, as a consequence, will be less vulnerable to hurt when you don't get it. To strengthen your inner resources, you need to discover and develop your value as a person with a chronic illness and evolve a life-sustaining purpose.

I realize personal development, whether you're ill or not, is a difficult prescription, but I'm talking about something important – your life fulfillment.

Editor's note: Some readers may question the inclusion of this chapter in the book because RLS cannot be considered a rare disorder since it is thought to be visited upon 12 million Americans. However, Dr. Flapan gives some sound advice for victims who may be unaware of RLS. Many people live miserable lives every day because they believe that what is troubling them is unique and something they have to endure alone. Letter after letter comes to the Foundation similar to this one:

I couldn't believe that there are millions of people out there who have this problem. I thought I was the only one.

Unfortunately we live in a world where the devastation of RLS is underappreciated. The RLS Foundation is dedicated to informing the medical world and the general public that RLS is a physical, treatable disorder.

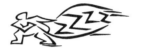

Chapter Two

Ways to Cope at Work and at Home

by Virginia N. Wilson

After the WHAT of my lack of sleep and the need for my crazy, jumpy legs to walk were diagnosed as restless legs syndrome (RLS), I set about to learn all I could about the disorder.

In 1986, the year of my enlightenment, there was little published about RLS except in a few medical journals of which I had no knowledge. Since I could not find the answer of WHY I had it, nor the answer to WHERE I got it, I concentrated on the WHO and the WHEN.

I soon discovered WHO may be attacked: any human being of any nationality, male or female, the highly educated and the barely literate, the rich and the poor, the over-weight and the thin, those ill with diverse ailments, and those well except for RLS. The victim may have inherited RLS from parents or perhaps be born with it, only becoming aware of it and suffering its devastation in later years. To pinpoint the true source of RLS is still a mystery, a sleep thief who indiscriminately chooses victims to be robbed of one of life's most important necessities – rest.

The WHEN included all ages: the very young, the teenager, the middle aged, and the old. It is very important for every RLS victim to read, learn about sleep disorders, and seek a credible physician. Sometimes the best doctor is one who does not understand RLS, but will listen, read your information, and want to help. Listening is a number one priority. If your doctor doesn't want to hear your tale of sleep deprivation or dismisses your woes as figments of your imagination, find another doctor. There are caring physicians who understand that even though sleep therapy has not been included in the medical curricula, sleep is of primary importance. Every day those doctors are reading and hearing messages of the need for proper diets and regular exercise, so they are beginning to suggest those areas of therapy. Now the media – TV, newspapers, magazines – are stepping in to inform the whole world that SLEEP is also a very important element of life – to date under-explored. Research is proving that sleep restores the natural immune systems of the body. The hows or the whys are still a mystery.

Until the medical schools teach our physicians how to understand the area of sleep, we RLS patients must fill in the gaps for our own well-being. Proper medication, tailored to the individual, makes life worth living, but until the day comes that RLS is thoroughly understood we will have to make do with makeshift daily living – called COPING.

Here is a list of ways to cope that I have compiled during my search for answers of how to live a fairly normal life in spite of RLS.

• MOST IMPORTANT: Do not try to hide your RLS movements; you only make them worse. Tell your family, your church friends, your card-playing buddies, your surgeon, nurse, dentist, hairdresser and anyone else who will be performing services for you. Have extra brochures to give out to help educate the world that RLS is a real and treatable disorder.

• Start your day with stretching leg exercises. In fact, this is a good way to end the day too. Always stretch before walking or doing aerobics. Gentle exercises should always precede any kind of activity involving muscles. Nerves and blood vessels get trapped in hard muscles and can't flow smoothly, sometimes causing cramps and pain.

• Take your medication as prescribed by your physician, but don't expect your pills to do more than they can do. If you feel the medication is not working well for you, be sure to report how it is failing you. Proper results of medication come from a good patient-doctor relationship. Keep a written record of sleep patterns and if you have more than one physical problem with specialists prescribing special medications for those problems, as well as over-the-counter aids, alert your RLS doctor to be sure your prescriptions are compatible. Don't try to "cut down" on the amount prescribed without a consultation.

• Take your medication BEFORE you need it. Anticipate a possible attack. Never leave home without your pill box! Avoiding the tremors is 100 times easier than trying to stop them.

• Sleep late in the mornings if you find that you sleep better then. The National Disabilities Act allows for flex time. Try discussing this with your boss if your work can be done later in the day.

• If you find that it is impossible for you to remain seated at a desk, explore the possibility of having your desk and computer raised to counter height. Have a matching tall stool to sit on now and then. Production goes up 100%, as it stops hopping up and running around. This requires you to stand once in a while and stretch now and then. In lieu of raising your desk, use a tall stand to hold a book or place a book stand on a high counter while you read.

- When attending a show or church, select a seat on a far side aisle so that you will not have to trip over ten pairs of feet murmuring "Pardon me" as you tiptoe out. One nice thing is that the sermon or the play looks and sounds the same from the back of the room.

- Find others who have RLS. Prodigy or CompuServe can help you track other RLS patients who have signed up with the National Organization of Rare Diseases. It is another way to hope and cope.

- Join an RLS support group. If one is not available, form one. Each one helping another is the way this all began. It is still is the best way to cope with this mystifying disorder.

If your RLS gives you trouble getting and staying asleep:

- Try to keep a regular schedule for your bedtime.

- Accept the fact that sometimes your legs will not allow you to rest. Do not lie in bed and fight. You may enjoy listening to Books on Tape while walking on a treadmill. The time flies, plus you catch up on the literature you probably didn't ever get around to reading. Or you might play solitaire, do household quiet chores, work on your computer, work on your hobby until restlessness subsides. Keep busy. Many report the importance of using the hands and the brain as a team to help calm the body. Be alert until the **quiet time** comes. Stop your activity and go back to bed at once.

- If you have trouble getting to sleep, try listening to cassettes or "white noise" machines with sounds of the ocean or rain to block out disturbances. Some find soft radio music helpful.

- Absolutely, when all else fails take a twenty-minute soaking, warm tub bath (a jacuzzi is even better). Not hot! Warm water soothes. Turn the radio to soft music while you're in the tub. Helps to make the time go faster. If you have no tub, or can't get down into one, stand in the shower and let the water gently pour over your back and legs. Soothing! Rub your legs and thighs with a brush or a cloth – gently.

• There are all kinds of pain-relieving lotions on the market if you need more help. The coolness of a menthol rub often quiets agitated legs. If your doctor prescribes medication for cramps or pain, take some before the pains get monumental. It takes a long time for the brain to get the message to quiet leg muscles.

• If your feet get cold, wear socks or use a hot water bottle.

• If the covers on your bed drag down on your toes to further complicate your sleeping possibilities, try a blanket holder that will keep the cover off your toes. If you can't find one retail, create one by bracing two pieces of plywood board, 27" by 16" (size for a single bed), at a 90° angle, so that the lower piece may slip under a mattress, leaving the upper piece to stand up-right for holding sheets and blankets. A slip or an old towel to cover the top half serves two purposes: masking the chilly roughness of the board and keeping the covers from sliding off the board.

• Avoid caffeine in the hours after noon. All the sleep experts declare this is most important. However, there are many Night Walkers who swear that a cup of regular coffee helps to quiet them and often take at least 1/2 cup sometime during the night. We don't take sides on this issue. Whatever works!

Night Walkers seem to respond to different methods of falling and staying asleep and often invent their own nightly sleep routines.

Chapter Three

Stop Muscle Abuse: Give Tender Loving Care to Your Legs
(with Illustrated Stretching Exercises)

by Virginia N. Wilson

Tired and weary of turning, twisting, and kicking while trying to fall asleep, RLS victims finally give up the fight and get out of bed to stand and march in place, left foot – right foot – left and on and on, hoping to relieve the jittery tenseness that has overtaken the legs, slyly and suddenly. Marching in place gives way to the beat of "Seventy-Six Trombones" which require steady pacing, the pounding of the feet one after the other or even jumping up and down, to stop the pulsing that demands attention. This is what some RLS patients say:

I could just beat my legs to a pulp.
I want to cut my legs off and throw them away
Sometimes I think I will wake up and find my legs in Hawaii.
. . . jumpy legs . . . I rock and roll for hours sometimes.
. . . tickling pain inside my bones causes me to beat on my thighs.

RLS sufferers wrote those words and sometimes victims do abuse their legs, not by hitting them or using an ax, but by overworking already oxygen-depleted muscles.

The RLS brain is like a marine drill-sergeant: "Stand at the desk if you can't sit down! Put weights on your ankles when you do leg lifts! Ride that bicycle harder! Ride it longer! Add tension to the wheel! Climb those steps higher! Walk farther! Run faster!"

RLS patients should not listen to their demanding drill-sergeant brains. They should not abuse their leg muscles that need to be protected from being over-worked. Outdoor exercises, walking, jogging or running, one or two miles at a time, are healthful and should be encouraged but they should be preceded by at least ten minutes of stretching the muscles to prepare them for expansion with fresh oxygen. All workouts should be followed by "cooling down" stretching. Frantic pacing in the night that turns into "dancing with Fred Astaire legs - not willingly" saps energy that is already strained to the breaking point. Start and end planned or unplanned activity periods with tender *stretching* care.

If your legs are severely abused, the blood vessels trying to wend their ways through knotted muscles are not able to supply oxygen properly. Nerves are trapped in tense and hardened tissue lacking elasticity which may result in painful cramps, both daytime and nighttime. The distress can become so severe that even walking is torturous. This might lead to the abandonment of any exercising resulting in added muscle distress.

In addition to prescribed medications for RLS and warm soaking tub baths, neuromuscular massage therapy may be helpful. Since both the nervous and the muscular systems are involved in the stress-tension-pain syndrome these hands-on treatments sometimes relieve tension distress. The muscles need to be softened and relaxed in order for the blood flow to return to normal. In fact, massage of any kind is relaxing and helpful especially if your "significant other" offers TLC for your RLS.

FOR THE ABUSED LEG MUSCLES

SIMPLE stretching exercises are imperative. One cannot hop to the health spa at one a.m., and isn't the whole idea at that time to get into a bed and sleep as quickly as possible? What is the purpose of the foot stamping in the first place? Isn't it to relieve the creepy, crawly sensations that spread faster and deeper into the muscles of the legs in order to sit down or to lie down for a rest? No matter what type of exercising the RLS victim finds helpful, especially in the middle of the night when everyone else in the household is asleep, whether it be riding the stationary bicycle, walking on a treadmill, using a stair climber, or just pacing around and around in the darkened house – hall, living room to kitchen and back – the leg muscles must be protected and STRETCHED. Every exercise program suggests a variety of ways to protect muscles before and after engaging in an active schedule.

DAILY EFFORTLESS STRETCHING FOR
EXERCISE OR RELAXATION:

Fig. 1

1. (Fig. 1.) Sit on the floor, back against a wall or bed. With a bath towel grasped in both hands and anchored in the arch of the foot, lift the leg upward, keeping the knee straight, stretch the back leg muscles. (You'll feel the stretching pull but you won't be injuring the abused muscles since your arms do **the work**, not the tightening of the leg muscles.) Take deep breaths with each lift to supply extra oxygen to your system. Repeat 15 times.

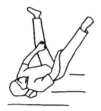

Fig. 2a.

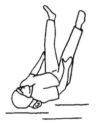

Fig. 2b.

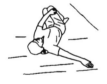

Fig. 3.

2. (Fig. 2a.) Lie on floor, place a small pillow under the head. Lift both legs up, straight at the knees, place hands on inner thighs, and gently move the legs by hand outward and then, (Fig. 2b.) with slight pressure on the outside of the thigh bring the legs inward slowly, without tensing any leg muscles. Hold the outward stretch for 40 seconds. Repeat 10 times.

3. (Fig. 3.) Still in prone back position put knees together and still using hands only push the legs from side to side. This pulls outer and inner muscles of the thighs. Do not use leg muscles for any movement. Take slow deep breaths to restore oxygen to aid in the recovery of the abused muscle. Repeat 10 times. These last two exercises may be done while still flat on your bed upon waking in the morning as an extra help to get the blood moving, to flex the muscles before you start your day. At 82, I sometimes find getting up from the floor mat a problem. Recently I began to do my floor exercises on my bed and it is easier on my old bones.

AVOIDING ABUSED MUSCLES

Develop a leg-muscle stretching program. Try these simple exercises and be surprised how they help painful legs. Do them several times a day: when you get up in the morning, at noon, in the afternoon while preparing dinner; or in evening when you want to watch TV and can't sit quietly. Even in the middle of the night when leg muscles cramp and demand a run, a short series of these exercises

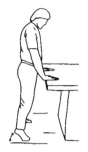

Fig. 4.

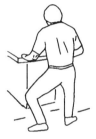

Fig. 5.

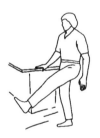

Fig. 6a.

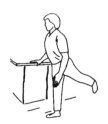

Fig. 6b.

may release the tension. If all else fails, a warm (not a hot) tub bath helps either before or after stretching.

1. (Fig. 4.) Preferably barefooted or in heelless slippers stand at a counter, bath or kitchen, with your feet 12 to 18 inches apart. Raise heels off the floor, then settle back on heels slowly, 10 times. Breathe deeply as you count a slow 1-2-3. You should feel the gentle pull on the anterior and posterior muscles of the thighs and lower legs, calf to toes.

(Fig. 5.) Remaining in the same position with the feet still placed 12 to 18 inches apart and firmly on the floor, squat gently (NOT deep -knee bends) slowly to stretch the inner muscles of the legs, 10 times. This routine may be done any number of times during the day and is very effective in avoiding or relieving leg cramps.

3. (Fig. 6.) Remembering the slow 1-2-3 count and still holding on to the counter for support, lift one leg straight out 10 times, then reverse the leg lift backward 10 times. Repeat with the other leg. You will feel the stretching of different muscles.

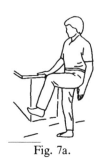

Fig. 7a.

4. (Fig. 7.) Next, bend the knee and lift the leg high in front with a 1–2–3 count for 10 times. Reverse: lift the heels high in the back toward the buttocks. Repeat the exercise with the other leg.

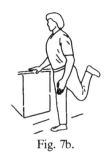

Fig. 7b.

5. (Fig. 8.) Put hands on wall at shoulder height, place toe of one foot close to the wall and position other foot as far back as possible keeping the heels of both feet firmly on the floor; bend the knee of the leg nearest the wall, and stre-e-e-e-etch the muscle in the other leg. Be sure to keep the back heel firmly pressed against the floor for the slow count 1-2-3. Repeat 10 times. Reverse the feet and stretch the other leg muscles. This may be done holding on to door frame and placing one foot against the door sill.

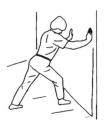

Fig. 8.

Drawings by Shawn Gallagher

These simple-to-do exercises may be done by almost anyone who is able to stand because they are gentle and the vigor may be controlled by the exerciser. They warm the legs and get the blood stirring into the leg muscles BEFORE and AFTER more strenuous forms of exercise or they may be used as the only set of exercises an RLS patient may be able to do. Even beneficial brisk walks should be preceded and followed by simple warm-up procedures. They will avoid a lot of knotted muscles which can turn into painful cramps. This should be done every time you do any kind of leg muscle exercising to avoid nerve and blood vessel entrapment.

(That condition can be extremely painful if allowed to develop to an abused, injured state. Untying entrapped muscles is not easy or painless!)

Then there are the old standbys of lying on the floor, or on a bed if there is a problem getting up off the floor, and lifting the legs one after the other – up and down, side to side, turning over and lifting the legs up in the back. Many RLS sufferers do these in the middle of the night out of desperation, often falling to sleep there on the floor after or during the back-leg lifts. Be sure to wear warm-up suits while doing these. If you do fall asleep you may wake up several hours later, stiff as a board, but sometimes the floor feels good and sleep creeps up suddenly. Call that putting the sleep thief to sleep.

Many people find exercising in water is helpful and attend classes at spas. This is especially preferred by those who suffer with arthritis, for the buoyancy of the water makes movement easier and less painful.

Remember whatever we do for our bodies to keep them healthy is important. Don't forget to stre-e-e-etch those easily abused leg muscles.

Restless legs may not shorten life but they lengthen nights.

Dr. Steincrohn

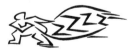

Chapter Four

Stop RLS Hospital Torture Time

by Virginia N. Wilson

Since RLS is a little known disorder, and until the whole medical arena has been alerted and trained, it will continue to create nightmare events like the ones experienced by many RLS sufferers. Letters pour in with horrifying experiences. RLS Hospital Torture time is greater than any fiction writer could dream up, but you need not let it happen to you.

Jeannie wrote about her May (1990) hip replacement:

*I could write a **horror story** about what I went through with my RLS. I was packed in ice, had a large foam pillow strapped to my legs to keep them apart. I was in horrible pain and I begged and pleaded to be let out of bed because my RLS was **terrible**. They gave me pills and nothing worked. My husband stayed with me night and day, rubbing my feet and back trying to get my legs calmed down.*

As soon as the IV came out I was let out of bed and it was the biggest relief of my life. The nurses had never dealt with such a problem, and they didn't know what to do. I really don't know how I ever got through those twelve days.

J. S., Livingston, Texas

I was sent to ER [hospital emergency room] with a breathing problem and RLS was bothering me much, so that ER doctor gave me four shots of tranquilizer – each one agitating me more until they had to hold me down on the table. I told them I had RLS, which meant nothing. My own doctor was out of town, so I just had to lie there on the torture rack.

F. P., Waterloo, Iowa

F.P. wrote another letter dated June 13, 1994:

After saying I'd never go through the pain of a total knee replacement, looks like I'll have to have the other one done. You mentioned in a newsletter that you had some suggestions about an RLS hospital stay, so I need to know all I can, especially since I was tortured with tranquilizers one time in an emergency room. After telling that doctor three times, he shot me three more times, each time making me worse and then said he was going to tie me down because he'd given me enough to knock out an elephant. I will appreciate any helpful information you can send.

These are samples of the many letters which describe the tortures experienced by patients because the doctors and nurses (and sometimes the patients themselves) are unaware of the devastating effect of RLS. The mission of the RLS Foundation is to inform those who work in the medical field how to recognize and better understand this disorder but at the same time to emphasize the importance of the patient's need to help assure that good care will be received.

This is my response to F.P.'s last note with a few hints that have worked for me.

Dear Fran:

So glad you told me about your upcoming hospital stay. First of all you need a positive attitude. Just remember you are going to be a guest of the hospital. Everyone is there to serve you and they really want to have a good report that you were happy about your time spent as a guest. Patients have rights and the hospital personnel is responsible for making your stay as pleasant as possible.

*This next part is the most painful: **strain your memory**. Examine all the negative things that happened during any bad experience of treatment you had in any hospital. Write them down so you won't forget any of them. Now study what you need to do to get everybody who might be handling you educated about RLS. No doctor or nurse wants to admit that he or she doesn't know about or is baffled by a disorder named RLS. We'll call it professional pride to hide the lack of knowledge. You just have to realize that RLS is still very much an unknown condition. YOU are responsible for educating a small area of the medical world about what to expect from **your** body.*

*First, talk to your doctor whom you trust – the one who oversees your RLS treatment. Enlist his or her help. **Tell exactly how you feel about going to the hospital.** Share your fears about being given shot after shot to quiet you. Share the dread of having to move your legs when you can't because they've been tied down. Make an emotional plea for your doctor to take an active part in your hospitalization – at least in the medication part by talking to the surgeon who will be wielding the scalpel.*

Take a brochure and a doctor packet (available to all Night Walkers) for the surgeon to read. Tell exactly what you told your regular doctor – how much you've suffered from those trying desperately to serve you. If the surgery is to be long lasting ask that your own doctor be present. It is comforting to know someone you trust will be there for you, if only for a short while.

*Request a meeting with the anesthetist. Also take a brochure and doctor packet with you. I will include that, too. THIS IS IMPORTANT. Those who give anesthetics often have never heard of RLS. **They like to be educated.** The one who worked on me said he had often tied people down when they thrashed about. He just didn't understand the compulsiveness of the condition. Discuss the proper* *anesthetic. I had an epidural which makes the legs numb. It is what they use for mothers having a C-section, so I felt it was safe, as they wouldn't give something too strong for a newborn baby. I told him to give me something at the last minute to put me to sleep so I wouldn't hear what was going on. I recalled that during two baby deliveries I could hear but couldn't speak or move. I have never forgotten those delivery room conversations. I didn't want listen to chit-chat this time.*

There is no need to have a bravado attitude and say you can stand anything! Let them feel a little sorry for you! It's time the medical profession knows that RLS is not a "funny disorder," in spite of its frivolous name. The doctors will respect you for having leveled with them.

I was allowed to take my medication prior to the operation with a bare sip of water. After the operation the anesthetist came to my room three times to be sure I was all right. When you confide in doctors they respond! I was maintained with an even level of epidural for several days until I was able to take by mouth the medication to control my legs.

Sometimes the physicians don't take the packets and information as readily as you would like, but don't be discouraged, they will learn in time. The nurses greedily snatch up the brochures (available free to Night Walkers). I took twenty with me and handed them out to every nurse who came in the room. I was surprised at how eager they were to learn about RLS. Those brochures disappeared like magic in no time.

My medical doctor had left word not to disturb me if I were sleeping, as I had a problem with that. No waking me up at 5 a.m. to wash my face. I had a private room, as I sleep on the edge of being awake all the time. Also I could play the TV whenever I wanted to have a bit of "companionship." I often keep my own TV on at night (light muted with several layers of chiffon scarves) in my bedroom with the voice down to a murmur, and it helps me sleep. Just a quirk of mine, I'm sure.

If you plan ahead and have doctors who will cooperate with you, your hospital stay will be pleasant. Letting them know ahead of time that you have an uncontrollable problem is most important.

Whatever the reason for your hospitalization, it is always important to advise your doctor about your RLS. Just days before "Sleep Thief" was finished, I was told by an ophthalmologist how important such information would be to him. "Removing cataracts, for example, can be much more difficult in RLS patients," he explained. The eyes often move just as the legs do and he would rather be prepared to deal with this by knowing in advance.

Best wishes for a speedy and pleasant recovery.

An added thought:

Being taken to the hospital emergency room is an altogether different story. I really hadn't thought of that until I had to call 911 one night for a friend who had a heart attack while visiting our house. The rescue squad came within a few minutes.

The medical technicians looked for a necklace or wrist medical tag. Finding none, they immediately started a flow of tranquilizer into his veins. I almost freaked out, as I knew what would happen to me if that were administered to me. I have violent reactions to most sedatives. After one shot I hit the ceiling and it takes six hours to calm me enough to sit down. I know that if I am sick and can't relate that information to emergency caretakers they will automatically go about with routine medicating unless they are alerted by a medical tag.

The very next day I ordered a medical alert bracelet and I put a card in my billfold giving instructions about what not to use on me. So take precautions if you have violent reactions. This is a most inexpensive way to protect yourself from emergency mishandling. Take the time to have such information made readily accessible and wear it always. You never know when you might need it.

Chapter Five

Networking

by Virginia N. Wilson

In August I received a note from Fran P. of Waterloo, Iowa, written shortly after she had moved into a retirement complex:

Dear Virginia,

I do love it here at The Village. Everyone is so kind and helpful. I really like this kind of living. The food is great too, but I just go to the dining room once a day. When I can't sit still I have my dinner sent up. Like tonight – I guess. I wonder how many miles I've walked the past twenty-four hours.

I met a gentleman here who also has RLS. I gave him all your letters and literature from the support group to read. He said he found them very interesting.

Another note from Fran came in December:

Dear Virginia:

The gentleman here who has RLS told me again yesterday that he just wanted to scream and cry for two hours last night, but it doesn't do any good to mention it because nobody knows what I'm talking about and they have their own problems. That's the way it is in a retirement community especially a lifetime care one.

In January I received a note from the gentleman:

Dear Mrs. Wilson:

I have been reading letters sent to the lady who also lives in the retirement center. As I also have the same problem, I noticed her when she moved in. I could easy see her problem . . . . I was diagnosed as having RLS but I also have an old back injury which makes it worse. I just have to live with it, as they don't know what more to do. I am a retired dairy farmer. Retired 10 years ago, I'm now 81 years old . . . .

G. S. Waterloo, Iowa

Fran's February note said:

G. stopped me after our monthly birthday party to say he wanted to meet my daughter, but I know what he really wanted was to tell me that he took the last information you sent him to his doctor and the doctor has prescribed medication for him. I was surprised when he said, "Now, I'm one of you. I joined the Night Walkers."

Two months later Fran wrote:

As I was walking the hall at eleven last night, I met Glenn who lives quite a ways from me on the first floor. He said he'd be up until three a.m. So – we suffer through the night while most residents are sleeping.

They both agree that having someone who understands the problems of suffering through RLS attacks helps. Just knowing someone is there who understands is important.

Networking! We can't cure RLS yet, but we can make it easier to bear. We are not always so lucky as to have a fellow sufferer live in the same building to share bad days or nights, so the alternative is to participate in a local RLS support group, which is a good way to help yourself. If there is none in your area, start one. Seek out a friend who has RLS and who wants to talk with a fellow sufferer to trade and share ideas that help.

This letter tells of what sharing information and understanding can do:

Just a short tale of how you have helped an RLS sufferer. I listen regularly to a local radio talk show – actually it is a mental health counselor giving advice. A woman phoned in to ask if the counselor knew of anything that her elderly mother could take to help her sleep. Then she went on to describe what I knew to be RLS (my husband suffers from it.). The counselor knew nothing of the syndrome or help for people with it. I immediately picked up the phone and called in to say what the syndrome was, the medicine my husband was taking for it, the name of your organization, etc. and gave the counselor my phone number. Two weeks later the elderly woman phoned me in tears. She had been to the doctor, received a prescription for the same medicine my husband takes, and just the night before had slept all night – for the first time in 40-some years! She was so thankful, and I was thrilled for her. You do work wonders! Thank you from me and my husband.

K. H., Omaha, Nebraska

That's the way this whole RLS Foundation began. A handful of bewildered night walkers satisfied our needs to share our distressing problem by letters and phone calls. Each of us felt very alone, isolated, and unable to change our lives. The thought that we might one time grow into a large national organization never entered any of our heads.

Today is a new day with the sun shining brightly enough to counter the night-time darkness that we dread. The spread of knowledge about RLS, through newspapers, magazines, radio, television, and word of mouth, has enlightened many thousands of people about this disorder. But we have many millions more to educate.

No longer are we a silent group of victims. We have an important voice in the medical world. The years of ignoring our pleas for help are over. We have been heard and our problem will be addressed. When? The wheels of change grind slowly, but we must press hard to have sleep disorders, including RLS, added to all medical school curricula. If any of you have clout with Congress, or with any medical school, please press forward for reform.

With all the publicity has come rapid growth for the RLS Foundation, and with the rapid growth has come the crying need for local support groups. Many of you write asking about networking in your area. Join an RLS support group. If one is not available, form one. Each one helping another is the way this all began. It is still the best way to cope with this mystifying disorder.

The purposes of the local support groups and the national Foundation are different:

• The local support group aids individuals who suffer from RLS by offering mutual physical and moral assistance to fellow victims through the exchanging of information and experiences. Smaller local groups can offer friendship on a one-to-one basis that the large foundation cannot provide. Local groups have a unique ability to work with local doctors and facilities to advance the effectiveness of the work of the Foundation.

• The Foundation works on the national and international fronts seeking to educate the general public and the medical world, including primary physicians as well as sleep specialists, that RLS is a physical and treatable disorder; to alert government agencies of the need for SLEEP RESEARCH (including RLS as a major sleep disorder in all studies); and to press for the inclusion of SLEEP studies, including RLS, in all medical curricula.

In order to be considered a part of the national network under the umbrella of the RLS Foundation, and using the name or the printed informational material, the Foundation requests that the founder, the organizer or facilitator of any RLS Support Group be a Night Walker who understands and supports the work of the National Foundation.

Realizing the importance of support groups the Foundation recently added a new member to the Board of Directors, Thelma Bradt of Bradenton, Florida, to assist with the starting of such groups.

The Foundation provides guideline packets for the forming of local support groups made up of those suffering from RLS. These guidelines, borrowed from other successful health groups, are only suggestions for possible members to discuss and grow with.

The Foundation furnishes printed materials such as brochures, stationery, and information sheets to hand out that may vary from time to time. However, the Board of Directors of the RLS Foundation is not responsible for any group's success or failure. The tasks of running the Foundation are too varied and complex to add local group management to the agenda.

The Foundation does not assume the financing of local groups. It may assist with some postage expenses to start a group and furnish the names of those living within a certain area who might want to participate on the local level. After the initial meeting it will be up to the group itself to decide how to meet group expenses.

The Foundation is always pleased to have local groups supporting and publicizing the work that is being done on the national level. Forming and keeping active any group is time consuming and sometimes exhausting, but the end results of knowing you are able to help others is worthwhile. Those of us who have worked long and hard making the RLS Foundation a reality would have it no other way.

The Joys of Being in a Support Group

by Thelma Bradt

Member of the Board of Directors of the RLS Foundation

Director in charge of RLSF Support Groups

"Misery Loves Company." How often we have heard this cliché. When attending a Restless Legs Syndrome Support Group, we discover the profound truthfulness of this statement. Certainly not many things are as miserable as being afflicted with RLS, and sharing this misery with others who know what you are talking about, if not a joy per sé, will do until something better comes along.

How much more lonely and isolated can we feel in the middle of the night, while walking the floor through a quiet, dark, sometimes cold house, with soft sounds of others sleeping peacefully filtering into our consciousness? We are left by ourselves to deal as best we can with what seems like a monster controlling our bodies. Alone with our own thoughts and feelings, exhausted from lack of sleep, unable even to sit and read or relax, desperation takes over. We become fearful. We cry. Feelings of hopelessness overtake us. We sometimes panic and scream out in our frustration at being unable to stop the creepy, crawly, prickly, sometimes painful feelings which necessitate our constant moving, making sleep impossible. Even our spouses and other family members, as compassionate and understanding as they may be, cannot possible know the misery we feel at such times.

Knowing that there are 12 million or so others "out there" somewhere, probably doing the same as you are, helps only minimally. How much better to actually have someone right there with you to talk to, to share with, to understand what you are feeling. But at one, two or three o'clock in the morning? Unless another family member living with you has RLS as well (which is possible, since this disorder is often genetic), and happens to be walking the floor at the same time, there is no one with whom you can talk and share.

Then one day you hear of a local support group, meeting for the purpose of discussing and sharing experiences and information regarding RLS. You attend. To your utter amazement, you discover the importance and joy of realizing that you have at last found others who suffer as you do. Ideas, information, feelings, and knowledge are shared with one another. You meet new friends – friends you feel comfortable calling between meetings and chatting with about your mutual miseries.

One might surmise that at a meeting of people with RLS and /or PLMS, you would find a group of fidgety, anxious, unhappy folks, grumbling and feeling sorry for themselves. Amazingly, this is not true. Except for the subject matter, a stranger in our midst would never know that we do, in fact, suffer all these aforementioned symptoms. Perhaps it is not amazing, but simply proves the point: getting together to share and support one another relieves these symptoms and provides a joy that reveals itself in smiles and laughter.

This is not to say there are not serious moments. Certainly there are many such times. It is at those times, however, when the full meaning of "support group" is apparent. There is something so fundamentally reassuring to hear others echo your feelings – statements like, "I have that, too" or "That's exactly what happened to me."

Hopelessness is replaced with hopefulness.

Perhaps the greatest joy in being a member of a support group is to learn that others are getting help! That we, too, can find help. We learn of ways to cope; of ways to alleviate the symptoms; of medications that work or don't work; and perhaps most importantly of doctors who know about RLS! Regarding this last point, it is mind-boggling to learn how many doctors have never heard of RLS, let alone know what can be done to treat it. It is through support groups we find members who have found a source of good medical help. For those who do not wish to go to a new or different doctor, there is information, including handouts, to take to their own doctors. So at the same time the members are discovering new information, so, too, are their physicians.

We receive assurance we are not crazy, that all these feelings are not "just in our heads." At the same time, we find relief in learning that although what we experience is just as painful as always, at least others have it, too – **we are not alone.** Our worst fears are proved false. We are not going insane; we don't have something no one's ever heard of; it isn't a hopeless situation – there **is help**. Yes, indeed, there is joy in being a member of a support group. The joy of sharing; the joy of being informed and informing others; the joy of meeting new friends; the joy of helping one another as well as ourselves. Together, we may be able to make a difference.

For more information please write: Thelma Bradt, 10287 Silverado Circle, Bradenton, Florida 34202.

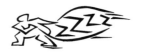

Chapter Six

Come Fly With Me!: Guidelines for Making Air Travel Pleasant

by Virginia N. Wilson

Any one who has RLS understands the torture of having to travel any distance by car, bus, or plane. Even a cross-town jaunt can turn into a nightmare of misery, so the mere thought of a long plane journey makes the RLS victim prefer to stay home.

RLS is a treatable, physical disorder. An RLS victim has certain rights to expect air travel to be at least tolerable as defined by the Americans with Disabilities Act. A number of airlines are providing disability service and more will do so when properly approached. If you are planning to take an extended trip, perhaps across the continent, these are suggested guidelines for a successful journey.

Step 1: As far ahead as possible, select the airline that best services the area you will be visiting and buy your tickets early. You will need copies of the tickets to go with your request for special services. If you are planning a very long trip, try to plan one or two stops along the way. It is a relief to go into the airport and walk around for some exercise to break the long ordeal of sitting in a plane.

Remember what you have endured during previous non-stop flights. Don't forget how you were sure you would be met by white-coated attendants with a straight-jacket at the end of your last journey. Recall how you had promised yourself that you would never, never fly anywhere, never go through that agony of being confined again. The airlines are wanting your business! They are willing to make your trip easier for you.

Up to the point of ticket purchase and credit card information you will be treated like any other traveler. Be sure to request an aisle seat near the rear of the plane, not the last seats as they tend to be a bit cramped with no head room at all. Ask for a seat five or six rows from the rear. Being next to the aisle in the back of the plane allows space for standing time. It's better to stand at the first wave of threatening movements before they overtake your legs completely. Being in the rear of the plane allows you to stand or walk a few steps without impeding any food services.

Step 2: Call the airline office for the name, address, and phone number of the person in charge of passenger services. You may have to make a long distance phone call to reach that person as it may not be part of the 800 ticket reservation service. It is worth the cost because the person on the other end of the line will probably not know about RLS.

No doubt you will be asked, "What is the restless legs syndrome?" You explain: RLS is a **disability** that sometimes causes severe involuntary movement of the legs which is relieved only by standing or moving. Offer to send a brochure from the Foundation to help explain the stress you sometimes feel. You might add that fortunately this doesn't occur all the time, but when it does it is real torture not to be able to stand. Then say that you will send along a letter from your doctor fully explaining your needs.

You will probably get an answer like this, "Yes, do that. I'll be very interested to learn about your problem and help you in any way.

Of course, we do have to follow the rules of safety, you understand."

Be sure and get the name of the person to whom you are speaking for your future reference. The call will be short, business-like and not expensive.

Step 3: Write a letter to your doctor (sample letter #1 at end of chapter). Several days later you will pick up the letter which Dr. Xyz had copied on his own letterhead stationery (letter #2).

Step 4: When the tickets arrive by mail, have copies made to go with the doctor's letter and your own (letter #3):

If you do not get an answer from the airline office of consumer affairs during the week before your departure week call the supervisor, or the person to whom you spoke earlier and ask about your RLS disability request.

Since the definition of RLS is still somewhat unknown, you will probably be told that yours was the first request from your foundation and it had gone into the legal department to be certain that the arrangements were made correctly. This is a new area of the American With Disabilities Act. However, thanks to the RLS Foundation the word is getting out that it does work. The letter arrives (letter #4).

Step 5: Check your medication before you leave home, in a purse or a pocket for the flight plus enough to last the whole time you will be gone. It is difficult to get prescriptions filled away from your home pharmacy. (One time in my rush to get to the airport on time I left all my medication on my dressing table and didn't discover it until late that night. I was 1,000 miles away and in a different time zone.) Also you need to be sure that you remain on your medication schedule, as it is especially important while on vacation to be assured a pleasant journey. Present your letters and tickets to the person at the gate of the boarding door. Explain your need for a last minute boarding. Be sure to have a number of the RLS brochures too.

They are free for the asking from the RLS office and they save a lot of explaining. Most stewards and stewardesses are interested, since they often see people with this disorder and don't know what to do.

Step 6: Remain about the area near the entry gate to get the last taste of freedom for your legs. A good tip: If you have a Significant Other with you, suggest an earlier boarding than your own to stow carry-on luggage so these can be in place at your seats. The stewardess will motion for you to come aboard as flight time arrives. With the flurry of passengers getting settled and buckling their seat belts you will find your aisle seat. (You will be walking among other late boarders who are scrambling for luggage space, opening one and then another overhead bin to find an empty one.)

Step 7: During the flight a stewardess may stop and ask how you are doing. You will notice being able to step into the aisle and stretch your legs now and then makes a difference. The location of your seat is important too. You will not be trapped in the middle of the plane where the refreshment carts roll by or other passengers are moving about or will you be crunched down trying to stand beneath the stored luggage.

Step 8: If you've booked your flight on planes that have short layovers, to avoid being cramped in a narrow space for a long time, you may deplane and return by telling your stewardess of your plan. I'm sure she will accommodate you. There are always others flying who complain of being confined too long. You will have time to look around the airport while having a few minutes to walk around and stretch. You'll feel refreshed for the next leg of the journey.

Step 9: Feel good. Even though you are not one to make public gestures of affection give your Significant Other a hug. After all, people will be giving hello and good-by kisses all over the airport. You can say, "I hope you don't care about making extra stops, Honey. So far the trip has been great!"

You'll hear an answer, "I remember how you cried on our last long trip. What a change!"

With one more short stop, you won't believe the captain's voice when he announces your final destination will be reached in fifteen minutes. The journey may take a little longer than a non-stop flight – but the difference!

Step 10: Letter #5: When you return home please do write a thank you note to High Fly Air.

Postscript:

I took a two hour plane trip this month and found everyone at the airport very helpful. I had not bothered to get any letters ahead of time but I did have my brochures handy. I reassured myself that I had taken my medication. I had an aisle seat. I had wheelchair service, as my legs are not up to these modern mega-airports. I gave out the brochures. Everyone seemed interested. I had no problems with flying this time. However, RLS is still a new "kid on the block" and we have much educating to do; but we have already made a dent in the real world. Now people do not laugh when I say "I have the restless legs syndrome."

More often I hear the reply, "You know, I think my grandmother [or cousin, or boyfriend] has that."

I smile and nod. Our message is getting out! I hope we will soon be able to make flying more pleasant so that we will no longer receive letters like this:

On plane trips I have to walk. Once I walked clear across the Atlantic.
M. G., Fort Pierce, Florida

From the desk of Nancy Jones

Date

Dear Dr. Xyz:

I wonder if you will help me with this request to High Fly Air regarding my need for special services under the Americans with Disabilities Act. I have already contacted Ms. C. Smith, the Supervisor of Consumer Affairs, so she is expecting a letter from you.

This is a part of the larger project to persuade all airlines to make similar accommodations to any RLS patient who presents a letter from his or her physician. Already we have had success with several airlines for our members. I am enclosing a sample of one reply. We are encouraging our members to use this service so they may travel in some comfort.

For your convenience I have included a suitable letter which you may have copied or amended in any way. When I send your letter with a copy of our tickets to Ms. Smith I will include one of the foundation's brochures, as RLS is unknown to her.

I know you are extremely busy but the foundation is trying to make travel for RLS victims more pleasant. Actually I dread my trip to the coast but I have to go to my father-in-law's 80th birthday and his family reunion.

Thank you so much.

Sincerely,

Nan Jones
Address
Phone Number

enclosures

Sample Letter #1

Ronald Xyz, M.D.
Family Practice
1700 Main St.
Terryville, USA 11111
Date

Ms. C. Smith,
High Fly Air, Supervisor of Consumer Affairs
PO Box 000
Anytown, US 00000

Dear Ms. Smith:

I am writing to ask that flight attendants assigned to planes on the attached itinerary accommodate my patient, Nan Jones.

Mrs. Jones has a neurological disorder called Restless Legs Syndrome which causes uncontrollable muscle spasms in the legs when sitting for long periods of time. While the muscle spasms are not life threatening, they cause serious physical discomfort and, once established, can last for several hours. Since Mrs. Jones should avoid sitting longer than 30-45 minutes, the condition is particularly acute during long airplane trips.

In keeping with the spirit of the Americans with Disabilities Act, I request that your attendants make a few simple accommodations which will enable my patient to travel.

1. Please allow Mrs. Jones to be one of the last passengers to board the plane.

2. Please be sure she is assigned an aisle seat, preferably toward the rear of the plane.

3. During flight, please allow her to stand frequently, perhaps in the galley area or in another space where she will not interfere with food and beverage service or create safety problems.

Thank you in advance for your efforts to accommodate my patient. I hope these precautions will head off the onset of muscle spasms which for this patient can last for several hours. Please feel free to telephone me if you have questions. Otherwise, I would appreciate your sending a letter to Mrs. Jones confirming that you agree to these precautions and that the appropriate flight attendants will be alerted to her needs.

Sincerely,

Ronald XYZ, M.D.

Sample Letter #2

From the desk of Nancy Jones

Date

Ms. C. Smith
High Fly Air, Supervisor of Consumer Affairs
PO Box 0000
Anytown, US 00000

Dear Ms. Smith:

I talked with you several weeks ago about the request for special services during my upcoming trip to the coast. While this effort by the airlines to accommodate RLS patients under the Americans With Disabilities Act is new, the foundation is finding that the service is successful, making traveling by plane pleasant instead of torturous. Up until now RLS patients have tried to avoid air travel if at all possible. The guidelines are offered by the *Night Walker* newsletter to encourage this quicker mode of transportation.

Enclosed please find several brochures to acquaint your staff with this disability. Included also is a letter from my doctor, a copy of our tickets and a sample letter from Fly Anywhere Airlines issued to Virginia Wilson which you may use as a guide for your own letter.

Thank you for your courtesy. We hope to be using airlines more often.

Sincerely,

Nan Jones
address

Sample Letter #3

HIGH FLY AIR
P. O. Box 0000
Anytown, US 00000

Executive Suite
Consumer Affairs

Date

Mrs. Nan Jones
address
city

Dear Mrs. Jones:

Thank you for providing the requested documentation regarding the Restless Legs Syndrome. We appreciate your selecting Fly High Air as your carrier, and we value your continued patronage.

This letter serves as confirmation that Ms. Nan Jones has provided medical documentation that she has a neurological disorder referred to as Restless Legs Syndrome. Mrs. Jones' concerns are that she will need to board the flight last, and that she will need to stand frequently.

Mrs. Jones has been advised, and indicated that she understands that there may be some situations that may impair our ability to permit her to stand. These situations include times that may result in a potential hazard to her safety such as take off, landing, turbulence, and when directed by a uniformed crew member.

Attached is a letter from Ms. Jones' physician. Please do all possible to accommodate Mrs. Jones' travel needs.

Sincerely

C. Smith
Supervisor, Consumer Affairs.

Sample Letter #4

From the desk of Nancy Jones

Date

Ms. C. Smith
High Fly Air, Supervisor of Consumer Affairs
PO Box 0000
Anytown, US 00000

Dear Ms. Smith:
I want to thank you and your splendid staff for my pleasant flight to and from Home Town and Far Coast this past weekend. Every consideration was given to me to ease my disability problems. The stewardesses were very co-operative and showed concern for my comfort.

Using the National Disability Act may make it possible for many others with the restless legs syndrome disorder to enjoy using frequent air travel instead of dreading and avoiding even necessary trips.

The foundation has prepared a paper advising others on how to use this service. Hopefully it will be as advantageous to your industry as it is to us individually.

Sincerely,

Nan Jones
Address

Sample Letter #5

Chapter Seven

How to Survive an Auto Vacation Trip

by Virginia N. Wilson

Does the following scene seem a replay of your last vacation?

"What do you mean stop? We haven't been gone from home thirty minutes and you want to stop already? We'll never get there."

"I know, but I have to get out and stretch my legs." We stop and get out of the car. Walk around, get back in, and we're on our way again.

Fifty miles down the road I am rubbing my legs together. Then I'm twisting in the seat, moving my legs, trying to quiet them. You say nothing but I know you're I thinking, *here we go again!*

"Better stop and have a walk break," I say, quietly.

We stop and I walk and walk. You sit and read the morning paper you had tucked beside the seat. We get back on the road.

"We'll never get to the campsite before dark if we don't make more time than this!"

"I'm sorry," I say as I concentrate on how beautiful the campsite will be. We will pitch our tent beside a lake so we can see the cleanness of the early morning dawn rise above the water. Even better, we will watch the moon reflecting its silver image across the lagoon: round full moon, with its trail of silver floating over the quiet, soothing water. You will have your jaunty fishing cap on, pulled down over your forehead testing the shadow the brim makes to protect your eyes. What could be better?

But my perfectly-painted vision fails to transform our to-the-lake journey, already halted at two-hundred and fifty miles, into a fun trip. We can't make it to the lake this first day after all. We stay in a motel. We eat the supper I had prepared for our first night beside the lake.

"I'm sorry we're so late but you know I couldn't help having to stop."

I hear your disappointed, wistful reply, "I imagine Bob is already out fishing."

I am angry at myself because I know I made the trip start out on a sour note. I knew, realistically, I couldn't get up at the crack of dawn and function after not sleeping the night before. I should have insisted on starting later. Well, I can't help that now. It's dark. The day's journey is over. We settle into the motel room where two queen-size beds await us. I marvel at your ability to lie down on the bed and immediately fall asleep. I listen to your gentle snore. Momentarily I am jealous of your quiet slumber while I am struggling, trying to rest. I am exhausted but sleep eludes me. The room is filled with furniture. I miss my big roomy house where I am able to roam around during the night. My jumpy legs take me into the bathroom where I turn the lights on and I play a game of solitaire (I never travel without playing cards) first on the counter, and then on the bathroom floor. Several times during the night, after too many games, which I almost never win, I open and shut the bathroom door, tiptoe around the room and peek out the shade-drawn window.

About five o'clock I see a tiny touch of pink in the sky. I lie down again, for perhaps the fourth try, and relax. Sleep creeps over me.

You pop out of your bed, immediately all rested, it seems, and ready for the day. Forgive me for not joining in your joyful exercise routine. For me, this is just another day to endure on the highway until we reach our destination where I will spend what is left of a week of nights in a tent. Do you wonder why I don't rejoice when you mention taking a vacation and going camping?

• • • •

Most family vacations involve the use of a car. All Night Walkers know what a nightmare riding in the car can be. When those twisty-turny "I-gotta-get-out-of-here" leg jitters begin, all the joy of a vacationing flies out the window. It is imperative that those riding with an RLS patient understand the torture that person endures in having to sit still while the legs want to run off by themselves. You may have to stop a dozen times to get out and walk around. If your legs have to move, take the time to move them. Wherever you are going will be there at the end of the road. True, you may take a day longer than your companion had figured but there is no need to suffer. Insist on taking your "walk" breaks.

Here are a few suggestions to help an RLS victim survive a journey by automobile:

• The number one rule is: Don't start your trip at the crack of dawn.

• Plan to stay in bread-and-breakfast lodgings, if possible, as you will have more room to walk around. Fortunately most RLS patients have sound sleepers for mates so your moving about probably won't be a disturbance. Put a deck of cards in your over-night bag so you can play a game of solitaire. If necessary, you can spread the cards out on the bathroom floor as I have done many times. Always warn others who might be using the bathroom with you that you might be restless in the night. On one trip we took with another couple we shared a suite. As usual I had trouble trying to sleep so I took my deck of cards and spread my game out on the bathroom floor. Some time later, in the quiet of the night, the door opened suddenly and slammed right into me. A sleepy, eyes-half-opened John, our vacation buddy, rushed into the brightly-lighted room, blinded with the glare, and fell over me. Fortunately neither of us was injured but there was much confusion and little sleep for any of us after that. We never forgot that night and have had lots of laughs over his shouting, "What the — are you doing in here on the floor?"

• If you aren't a solitaire-player, try carrying a folding stand to hold a book high enough for you to read while standing (and perhaps marching) in place. You can always read in the bathroom to keep the light out of your partner's eyes.

• Take along your tape player and earphones and listen to books you have wanted to read.

• If you are on your own for vacation and can choose your day's activities, try to arrange sight-seeing after a leisurely morning breakfast. You can't see and do everything so pick out the best and thoroughly enjoy it. Being exhausted is no way to begin or to end a vacation. Just traveling from here to there takes a lot of energy. If you are on a tour, there is really nothing to do but go with the flow. I have had to stop joining with others on bus tours, as the early morning calls and long periods of sitting became too much for me to handle.

• Try to avoid making appointments early in the day. I shudder at the thought of a 7 or 8 a.m. meeting, as I am usually just getting into my deep sleep for the night about 5 or 6 o'clock. Of course at conferences, early breakfasts seem to be the order of the day. The powers-that-be set the hour and there is no choice. My heart goes out to all of you when you cannot control the time frame. With my daily appointments I try for late morning or early afternoon. Most of us afflicted with RLS need that extra time to catch up on all the hours we miss during the night.

• Once in a while during a meal, especially while dining in a restaurant, you may find it necessary to get on your feet (or scream!). It's time to stand beside your chair and march quietly in place as your legs cramp and grab at you. Put a small amount of food on a saucer, carry it with you, and continue to eat. When the waitress says, "I understand. I get leg cramps too," SMILE, nod, and go on eating. The first time this happens, your dinner partner may be embarrassed and look faint. Go on talking as though nothing is wrong. Suddenly your legs will quiet. Sit down and do not apologize. Your legs had the fit and they don't talk.

• Some Night Walkers write that they do not experience RLS symptoms while driving a car. I do not do any long distance driving, as I mentioned in the chapter, "Are You a Danger to Yourself and Others?" I seldom have attacks when I am driving around town. However, the few that I have experienced were frightening. I always put my car in park while waiting for a red light to change. I certainly don't want to suddenly jerk into a car in front of me, either standing still or moving.

• Sometimes some of these hints simply do not apply. For instance, Laura, one of our Night Walkers, and her husband went on a photographic African safari. After Jeep-roaming over the wild lands, night approached, and they stopped to make camp and sleep in the tent provided by those in charge. Laura's legs didn't know they were in the wild country. They demanded a walk. For two nights she wandered into the dark camp area, walking around and around the campfire. On the second night the safari leader saw her in the flickering flames and demanded that she return to her tent for safety because lions, tigers, rhinos, and even crocodiles often lurked in the dark shadows. After that she remained inside the tent all night. Night hours crawled, seemingly endless. She prayed for the sleep angel to come and dazzle her with some magic sleep-dust. But there was no angel. As night after night she stood, somewhat bent over, beside her cot and marched in place, she kept reminding herself that dawn would come and she would survive. She coped by thinking of all the wonderful sights and all the wild animals that she would be able to snap photos of the next day. She repeated over and over the Night Walker's words, *cope and hope*. She knew the sun always rises . . . even in darkest Africa.

On the home front we are always looking for ways to solve a problem – and certainly the inability of one member of the family to ride in a car is a grave problem. Jack solved our travel woes by having a high top put on a second-hand Chevrolet conversion van. It has a folding side door with two small steps which make it easy for me to climb into the rear part of the van where there are two large upholstered bucket seats. We had the top made high enough for me to stand straight up in front of the bucket chair behind the front passenger seat. I have found that being able to stand whenever the creepy-crawlies start to tickle my legs actually stops attacks before they start. I fasten the safety belt across the front seat and hold on to it with my left hand. With my right clutching a hanger attached to the frame of the van I am fairly secure leaning against the heavily padded front chair seat. Of course Jack doesn't drive seventy miles per hour or do lane changing while I stand, so there is no lashing about for me. Actually I usually stand less than five minutes before my legs quiet. We do get out and walk quite often, however. We drove up to Raleigh to visit the Guthries and my journey was pleasant and certainly do-able and a great improvement over driving up there in our sedan.

We know this is not a perfect answer. When I announced what we had done, we had a number of calls and letters cautioning that this plan is not safe because I could be catapulted over the front seat into the windshield if I didn't wear some kind of safety belt. I do have a harness in the back seat which I wear while I am sitting in the chair but have to undo it to stand. So far this has worked well but we are working on an easily attached safety harness to use while I stand. That's our next project.

Bob Guthrie decided to try a different method to make travel possible for Pickett. I asked him to write down the details of installing an exercise bicycle in the back of a van. This is his letter to me and I'll share it with you:

Dear Virginia:

Let me try to tell you how I outfitted a minivan with the exercise bike. Pickett and I had been looking at a large van, the kind with an extended top. We knew of other RLS sufferers who had bought such vans and rigged up a method for the suffering spouse to stand up and walk in place when the RLS problem arose. We were not enthusiastic about this approach. Some talk about RLS patients using exercise bikes, seeing a recumbent exercise bicycle at the local YMCA, and a conversation with some minivan owners led me to try the approach we eventually adopted.

Once we determined that pedaling would relieve the RLS (you should check this before venturing further), I began looking for an exercise bike and at minivans. After considering a lot of vans, we settled on the General Motors minivan (the Chevrolet Lumina, Pontiac Transport, or Oldsmobile Silhouette style). I have a client who owns an Olds dealership so we purchased the Oldsmobile version although any of the others would work.

Here are the reasons we chose this style van: 1) it has three rows of seats, 2) the third row has bucket seats, 3) the seats are extremely easy to remove and reinstall, requiring no tools to do so. This van also has road feel more like a regular car than any of the others. This was important since I use it as my business car. I think a Toyota Previa van would work, but it does not have a bucket seat in the third row. I also believe that a GMC or Chevrolet Suburban could be used, but they are more expensive and would require more custom work.

I purchased a very simple exercise bicycle, an Ergomaster. It uses a flywheel and a brake to vary resistance. I have seen similar ones with different brand names. I removed the handlebars and seat and built a wooden plate with drilled holes so it could be attached to the seat-mounting brackets in the van. The front forks of the bike fit into the plate. I use a screen door chain and turnbuckles to hold the bike to the plate. The plate is bolted to the floor of the minivan via the seat brackets with some hook bolts which I purchased from the local hardware store. The bike sits behind the driver's seat. Pickett sits in the third row seat and pedals in a recumbent position. For more details see the sketch below.

P. S. There is an added advantage in that we can ship the bike ahead of us and rent a GM minivan to do some touring.

Bob Guthrie

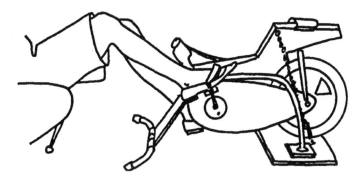

Marilyn Taylor

SECTION VI

The Past, the Present, and the Future of the RLS Foundation

Chapter One

Chronological Review of Restless Legs Syndrome

by Virginia N. Wilson and
Jeanne Schell, Member of the Board of Directors of the RLS Foundation

1672 oldest description of the syndrome written in a Latin manuscript by the British neurologist, Thomas Willis.

1685 Latin manuscript first published in English.

1695 second edition of English translation published by Willis.

1774 German physician aroused little interest when he dismissed the symptoms as being "hysterical"or "neurasthenic."

1861 article written by a German neurologist, Wittmaack, labeled syndrome "anxiety tibiarum," a form of hysteria.

1880 Beard, 1913 Bing, and 1923 Oppenheim mentioned *anxietas tibiarum* in writings.

1936 Code and Allen of the Mayo Clinic reported three cases of neurosis involving legs.

1940 detailed description of RLS published by Mussio Fournier and Rawak and again in 1947 terming it "paresthetic restlessness of the extremities."

1943 Allison, a sufferer himself, first to note the involvement of involuntary muscles jerks, termed the disorder "leg jitters."

1945 Dr. K. A. Ekbom coined the name "restless legs syndrome" in a series of comprehensive Clinical Studies (123 pages of his studies from the Neurologic Service of the Serafimer Hospital, Stockholm). In some literature, especially European, RLS is known as Ekbom's Syndrome. The Ekbom Support Group in England is an association similar to our RLS Foundation of the United States.

1947-1953 reports from French school (Bonduelle and Jolivet) suggested a defect in the circulatory disturbance in lumbar spine as a possible cause.

1949 Italian Tuvo wrote of involuntary muscular jerks accompanying restlessness.

1955 Dr. MacDonald Critchley, a British neurologist, published an article in a New York City "Medical Journal" quoting from the second edition of Willis' book printed in 1695.

1961 Israeli Bornstein suggested the disorder caused by defect in muscular tone.

1962 Dr. Elio Lugaresi and colleagues of the University of Bologna, Italy, added to the description of RLS by showing that involuntary kicking movements occur during sleep.

1960-70s Research seems to have been sporadic. Interest picked up after 1980.

1986 A marvelously complete report appeared in 1986 in the *American Family Practice Journal* by Dr. Gary N. Fox of Boise, Idaho. He made most specific differential diagnoses between true

Restless Legs, nocturnal myoclonus, cramps, hypnic jerks, and other similar conditions. At the same time members of our own Medical Advisory Board, Drs. A. Walters, W. Hening, S. Chokroverty and N. Kavey, as well as the group of Dr. Jacques Montplaisir from Montreal, Canada, began publishing articles in medical journals about RLS and myoclonus, including appropriate medications.

1990s It is encouraging to know that between 1990 and 1995 the National Library of Medicine indexed nearly 200 articles in English on RLS appearing in medical journals from Australia to Romania. There were more in other languages. Emphasis on worldwide cooperation of the study of RLS was demonstrated by the International Symposium on RLS held in Florence, Italy, May 1994, organized by Drs. Walters and Hening and the formation of the International Restless Legs Syndrome study group under their leadership.

• • •

From 1685 RLS has traveled a long and torturous road for recognition. Today it is acknowledged to be one of the most under-appreciated disorders in the medical sleep world and many Sleep Centers are adding the treatment of RLS to their agenda.

Since approximately one third of the human life span is relegated to sleep, the RLS Foundation and other sleep disorder groups such as the National Sleep Foundation, are working toward the goal of having all medical schools include the study of sleep and sleep disorders in their curricula. Naturally our RLS Foundation is pushing for RLS to be a part of those studies.

To bring research of these past three centuries up to date, it should be noted that there has been progress made in the study of appropriate medication but unfortunately the etiology of RLS is still a mystery. There are many hypotheses of the cause of this strange-acting disorder but so far none has been able to reveal the birthplace of the sleep thief.

The ultimate goal is finding the cause of and the cure for this devastating disorder through future scientific studies.

Author's note: Since caffeine is thought to aggravate RLS it is interesting that coffee, tea, and chocolate were introduced into Europe in the 1600s.

According to the *World Book Encyclopedia*, the drinking of these hot beverages became very popular and fashionable throughout the northern parts of the continent at that same time. Today Americans use more coffee and chocolate than any other people, with German, English, French, Dutch, and Swiss coming in close. Since many of our Night Walkers have ancestries rooted in these Northern European nations there may be some clue as to the etiology of RLS hidden within our historical pasts.

Chapter Two

The History of the Restless Legs Syndrome Foundation

by Virginia N. Wilson

Before plunging into a New World of RLS Recognition, it is time to think back to how this all began. In 1990 Oron F. Hawley of Escondido, California, exchanged letters with eight fellow RLS sufferers, including Jeanne Sissell, Roberta Sivori, Ben Struder, Jo Madden, Mar Mathna, Sheila Connolly, Sherry Bose, and Virginia N. Wilson, whose names he acquired from the National Organization for Rare Disorders (NORD). These letters shared ways to cope with RLS including the trial and errors of medications, any therapy from bananas to red hot pepper liniment. Best of all each one learned he or she was not crazy, not imagining sleep problems, and was not the only person in the world with legs that could not rest. A truly great message for all of us even today.

Being past ninety, Hawley withdrew as editor and Virginia N. Wilson volunteered to do the newsletter, *The RLS Night Walker*. She designed a query sheet to record medical history and family background as a requirement for becoming a part of the RLS Support Group.

By February 1991, 32 queries had been filled out by Night Walkers. Good, sharing friends sent stamp money as the project became rather expensive for Oron and Virginia.

In the February 1992 compilation of query facts of 62 Night Walkers a pattern of childhood RLS began to form. The words "growing pains as a child" written in the margins or on the back of the query sheets were noticeable. When the first 100 queries were tallied they were sent to Dr. Walters and he began a detailed study of RLS in childhood.

The need for a non-profit status became apparent. In September, 1992, the Articles of Incorporation of the Restless Legs Syndrome Foundation, Inc. were completed. The first Board of Directors consisted of Tim Byrne, president; Pickett Guthrie, treasurer; and Virginia N. Wilson, secretary. Hawley declined any post. A bank account was opened January 2, 1993, in Raleigh, North Carolina, with a gift of $1,000 from Elmer E. Hartgerink. The Directors approved the Medical Advisory Board (MAB), selected in February 1993 by Dr. Arthur Walters, which included Chairman Dr. Walters, and Drs. Wayne Hening, and Sudhansu Chokroverty.

April 28, 1993, new members of the Board of Directors were nominated and accepted: Sheila Courage Connolly, Elmer E. Hartgerink, Lester C. Sartorius, Jeanne M. Schell, Juanita W. Therrell, and Carol Upchurch Walker. Added to the MAB were Drs. Richard Allen, David Buchholz, Bruce Ehrenberg, Neil Kavey, and Joseph F. Lipinski, Jr. The final draft of the first brochure was approved by the MAB. The directors accepted the official logo of the shattered RLS initials.

The annual telephone conference meeting of the RLSF Board of Directors, September 28, 1993, elected Elmer E. Hartgerink Chairman of the Board. Pickett Guthrie was appointed Executive Director. A fee of $25 for a subscription to *RLS Night Walkers* newsletter was set. The Oron Hawley Scholarship was created to include hardship RLS patients unable to pay.

In January 1994 the first support group was established in Seattle by Juanita Therrell. Soon after came groups in Baton Rouge, Louisiana, by John Williams and in Fort Myers, Florida, by John Lingl.

March 1994 added three doctors to the MAB: Dr. June Fry, who at that time was President-elect of the American Sleep Disorders Association (ASDA), Dr. Ralph Pascualy, and Dr. Daniel Pichietti.

At the April 1994, annual telephone-conference: additions to the board of Directors were Robert M. Balkam and Martin Brinkley, who offered to serve as the legal adviser for the Foundation. President Tim Byrne's resignation was accepted. Chairman of the Board Hartgerink appointed Carol Walker, Pickett Guthrie, and Wilson to nominate a new President.

April 28 the Foundation had its first taste of legal problems with a misprint in the April newsletter. A simple error escalated into a costly, but educational experience. Hours of work and reprinting and postage that ran hundreds of dollars made the need for legal insurance foremost in many of the directors' minds. Guthrie and Brinkley secured liability insurance for the Foundation officers and directors.

Gifts to the Foundation: $5,000, Eloise Upchurch, mother of Carol Walker. Grants of $10,000 by Harry Le Bien, representing the Louis and Virginia Clemente Foundation, and two $1,000 grants to the RLS Foundation for educational purposes by DuPont Pharma were used to fund the RLS booth at the APSS annual meeting in June.

The first international symposium on RLS, held in Florence, Italy, in May 1994, was organized and chaired by Drs. Walters and Hening.

Along with Drs. Hening and Walters, Drs. Allen and Buchholz participated in the presentations.

Many firsts for the RLS Foundation occurred during the June week of the Association of Professional Sleep Societies (APSS) convocation of 1994 which proved to be a good opportunity for educating people who work with troubled sleep victims:

• first booth at a major medical meeting

• first symposium at APSS on RLS led by Dr. Richard Allen

• first meeting of the Board of Directors and the Medical Advisory Board. A dinner attended by Directors Hartgerink, Guthrie, Balkam, Connolly, Schell, and Walker joined Drs. Allen, Walters, Hening, Ehrenberg, Chokroverty, Fry, and Pichietti.

• first invitation to attend a work shop of the National Institute of Health (NIH).

• first recognition of RLS by invitation to become a member of the Patient Advisory Council of National Sleep Foundation.

At a called phone meeting June 30, 1994, Robert Balkam was elected President of the RLSF Board of Directors.

July 1, official national RLSF office opened, LeNoir Thackston, manager, 304 Glenwood Ave, Suite 6, Raleigh, North Carolina 27603

The September issue of the *Modern Maturity* magazine published the article, "Night Walkers" by Robert Yoakum which resulted in over 30,000 inquiries. This added to the interest generated by the article written by Jack Broom for the *Seattle Times* which had appeared during the year in many major newspapers crisscrossing the U.S.A. and Canada. Numerous other publications, such as the *Johns Hopkins Newsletter* and *Special Edition of Harvard Health Letter,* contributed to a national and international awareness of the RLS story.

In August 1994 Dr. Frankie Roman and in October Dr. Lawrence Scrima joined the MAB.

During January and February 1995 John B. Williams, James McNichol, Thelma Bradt, and Willard Hayes accepted places on the Board of Directors. Bradt was appointed chairman of the RLS Support Groups.

Pickett Guthrie and Dr. Richard Allen represented the RLS Foundation in Baltimore, January 1995 at the NIH strategic planning retreat attended by representatives of thirteen sleep disorders organizations. The primary purpose was to gather input from the participants to help assess trends and needs that will impact the future recognition and importance of sleep. This was an important step for the acceptance of RLS as a major disorder in the world of sleep medicine.

Juanita Therrell and Dr. Ralph Pascualy represented the Foundation at the Annual meeting of the American Academy of Neurology (AAN) in Seattle, Washington, March 1995. Drs. Walters and Hening made presentations at a scientific platform session. Dr. Sudhansu Chokroverty chairs the Sleep Section of the AAN, Dr. June Fry is secretary, and Dr. Hening is Editor of the Sleep Section of the AAN newsletter.

In May and June 1995, new doctors added to the MAB included Philip M. Becker, M.D.; Christopher J. Earley, M.D., Ph.D.; and J. Steven Poceta, M.D.

The American Sleep Disorders Association (ASDA) met at the Opryland Hotel in Nashville, Tennessee, May 31 to June 4, Dr. June Fry, President for the '95-'96 period. Dr. Allen chaired a course on RLS and PLMS with a panel of RLSF doctors: Walters, Hening, Buchholz, and Earley. Drs. Picchietti and Walters presented a Poster on the study of RLS in parent-child pairs.

The annual joint dinner meeting of the RLSF Directors and the MAB in Nashville June 1, 1995, was attended by Board members Hartgerink, Balkam, Guthrie, Wilson, Bradt, Sartorius, Schell, Walker, Williams, and Yoakum. Members of the MAB attending were Drs. Walters, Allen, Earley, Ehrenberg, Fry, Hening, Picchietti, and Roman.

Robert H. Waterman joined the Board of Directors in October 1995 and Dr. Richard L. Levin joined in January 1996.

The annual meeting of the RLSF was held at the Sheraton-Washington Hotel on May 30, 1996. The joint dinner meeting of the Board of Directors and the Medical Advisory Board was held at the same hotel on May 31, 1996. Sheila Connolly was elected President.

The work goes on, day after day, to ensure the survival of the RLS Foundation. Under the care of Thelma Bradt the number of support groups has grown to thirty with inquires for help to form such groups coming in weekly. This phenomenal growth is proof that victims and researchers working together can educate the medical world and the general public. Now we mail out 4,500 copies of each issue of the *Night Walker* newsletter to seventeen nations. Each printing increases that number. The address of the Restless Legs Syndrome Foundation, Inc. is 304 Glenwood Avenue, Suite 6, Raleigh, North Carolina 27603.

But it must never be forgotten that no matter how large the Foundation grows EACH NIGHT WALKER IS IMPORTANT. Coping and hoping, caring, and sharing makes life worthwhile.

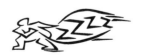

Chapter Three

Looking to the Future Through My Crystal Ball

by Virginia N. Wilson

Today RLS is recognized worldwide. Long neglected and ignored by the medical community, RLS is being discussed and studied by researchers, par excellence, at conferences in many countries. Members of the Foundation's Medical Advisory Board are speaking before gatherings of directors of sleep disorder centers and neurologists. In the near future the program will expand to include gynecologists, pediatricians, anesthetists, physical therapists, and nurses. The field is unlimited and as the term "RLS" becomes more familiar to laymen so will it become more important for medical care-givers to become informed. I predict that in time medical schools will include the study of RLS in their curricula.

The devastation of the deprivation of sleep has not been adequately explored. The major causes of the lack of sleep need more studies to determine how many millions of dollars are wasted each year by those unfortunate ones who search in vain for help. The television screens are full of advertisements proclaiming cures for insomnia. Insomnia, or temporary inability to rest properly, affects a large portion of the population infrequently but RLS unrelentlessly attacks its victims every night. No human body, constantly deprived of rest, can work at peak level, nor avoid becoming a safety threat to themselves and others in the home, the workplace, and on the road. Over and over again tests have proved that dexterity of mind and body are destroyed without regular renewal of energy through sleep. Like the engines of automobiles, the human body cannot run without constant refueling no matter how fancy the design may be.

Palliative medications are not the answer. Another prescription to replace the one that has worn out its strength in RLS victims is not the answer. The answer lies within the question: "Why?" Why does RLS strike some and not others? Why does it often affect generation after generation? Why does it leave no visible evidence but acts like a thief in the night to destroy the body and even the soul of its victims making living a hell on earth, driving some to the final act of desperation, suicide? "WHY?" is the question to be addressed and answered. The etiology of RLS must be one of our most important concerns. The RLS Foundation, now and in the future, will take an active lead in promoting partnerships between all sleep organizations, the government, university researchers, and pharmaceutical companies to explore this mystery.

I believe that some of the studies being done now by research scientists will solve this puzzle. Why do I believe that? Because from the beginning this group has been blessed. All of our needs have been met, often before we even knew of the requirements. All the work that has been put into the organizing and advancing this Foundation could not possibly be an exercise in futility. The purpose is positive. The goal is achievable. The prize is waiting to be found. This discovery may not help me in my advanced years, but think of the joy it promises for the other millions of people waiting for the good news! What a glorious future.

But while the Foundation will be ever watchful for opportunities to further research, the original concept of this Foundation must never be lost. Patients, victims in the large army of suffering people, need help now – today, tomorrow, and all the days to come. Too many still need to discover and to understand that RLS is a real, physical, treatable disorder and that it is not a figment of the imagination. Indeed it is a serious problem and not something for doctors, family, or friends to laugh about, to ignore, to jeer.

Delivering that message must continue. Until RLS is a known phrase, known and recognized by the general public and the medical world, the educational goal must continue to be number one on the Foundation's agenda. Our children and our grandchildren should not suffer as our generation and past generations have – in silence and ignorance.

The message within that crystal ball is

CONTINUE THE FOCUS ON RLS!

APPENDIXES

Appendix 1

Biography of the Author

Virginia N. Wilson
co-founder and secretary of the RLS Foundation
First Editor of *RLS Night Walker*

Virginia N. Wilson was born in Danville, Illinois, in 1913 and married Jack F. Wilson in 1935. Together they owned and operated The Danville Floral Company and Wilson's Hobby Shop until retiring to Florida in 1976.

While a florist, Virginia authored a syndicated newspaper column on bridal customs and holiday decorations. She has published a book of poetry, *Medal 1985, a collection of poems and photographs.* A number of her poems and short stories have appeared in both popular and literary magazines. Her color photographs and articles of travels in foreign lands have been featured in newspaper travel sections. She has been a reader-editor for *Kalliope, a journal of women's art,* and an active member of the National League of American Pen Women, North Florida Writers, and the Florida State and the National Poetry Societies.

After suffering a lifetime of sleeplessness, Virginia was diagnosed as having RLS in 1986. Four years later she joined with Oron Hawley and seven other RLS victims in a round-robin letter exchange which became the *RLS Night Walker Newsletter* with Wilson as editor, secretary, printer and mailer. In 1992 she began working with Arthur S. Walters, M.D. and compiled some of the data now being used for research projects.

Wilson recognized the need to reach the estimated 12 million untreated RLS sufferers. In January 1993, with Pickett Guthrie of Raleigh, North Carolina, as co-founder, the Restless Legs Syndrome Foundation, Inc. became a reality. Growing from the original eight, the Foundation now sends 4,500 copies of each newsletter to a world-wide mailing list.

In addition to the duties as secretary of the Foundation and member of the Executive Committee, Wilson edited the *RLS Night Walker* until 1994 and is now a contributing editor to the newsletter with the *Letter from Virginia.* Since 1991, Virginia has devoted full time to writing RLS informational literature from which the book, *SLEEP THIEF, restless legs syndrome,* evolved.

Appendix 2

Text Contributors

David Buchholz, M.D.*
Department of Neurology
Director of Outpatient Services
Johns Hopkins
Baltimore, Maryland

Giorgio Coccagna, M.D.
Clinica Neurologica
Universitá di Bologna
Bologna, Italy

Bruce L. Ehrenberg, M.D.*
Department of Neurology
Tufts University-New England
  Medical Center
Boston, Massachusetts

Mark Flapan, Ph.D.
Founder of Scleroderma Federation
  Tri-State Area
Author of articles for NORD, Re:
emotional effects of chronic illnesses.

Wayne A. Hening, M.D., Ph.D.*
Department of Neurology
Robert Wood Johnson Med. School
Univ. of Medicine and Dentistry of
  New Jersey
New Brunswick, New Jersey

Alan Kanter, M.D.
Vein Center of Orange County
Irvine, California

Elio Lugaresi, M.D.
Clinica Neurologica
Universita di Bologna
Bologna, Italy

Jacques Montplaisir, M.D.
  Ph.D., FRCP
Centre d'etude du Sommeil
Hôpital du Sacré-Coeur
Montréal, Canada

Ralph Pascualy, M.D.*
Sleep Disorders Center
Providence Medical Center
Seattle, Washington

Daniel Picchietti, M.D.*
Pediatric Neurology Sleep Center
  Carle Clinic
Urbana, Illinois

J. Steven Poceta, M.D.*
Neurologist
Scripps Clinic and Sleep Disorder
  Center
La Jolla, California

Frankie Roman, M.D.*
Director, Center for Sleep Disorders
Massillon, Ohio

Lawrence Scrima, Ph.D.*
Sleep Alertness Disorder Center
Aurora, Colorado

Claudia Trenkwalder, M.D.
Neurologische Klinik
Max-Planck Institute for Psychiatry
Munich, Germany

Arthur S. Walters, M.D.*
Department of Neurology
Robert Wood Johnson Medical School
New Brunswick, New Jersey and
  VA Medical Center, Lyons, New
  Jersey

*RLS Foundation Medical Advisory Board

Text Contributing Members of the RLSF Board of Directors

Appendix 3

Publications Relating to RLS
by Arthur S. Walters, M.D. and
Robert M. Balkam, Past-President of the RLS Foundation

Akpinar S. "Treatment of Restless Legs Syndrome with Levodopa Plus Benserazide." *Archives of Neurology.* 1982; 39:739.

Akpinar S. "Restless Legs Syndrome: Treatment with Dopaminergic Drugs." *Clinical Neuropharmacology.* 1987; 10: 69-79.

Aldrich MS, Shipley JE. "Alcohol Use and Periodic Limb Movements of Sleep." *Alcoholism, Clinical and Experimental Research.* 1993; 17:192-6.

Allen RP, Kaplan PW, Buchholz DW, Earley CJ, Walters JK. "Double-Blinded, Placebo Controlled Comparison of High Dose Propoxyphene and Moderate Dose Carbidopa/levodopa for Treatment of Periodic Limb Movements in Sleep." *Sleep Research.* 1992; 21:166.

Allen RP, Kaplan PW, Buchholz DW, Walters JK. "A Double-Blind, Placebo Controlled Study of the Treatment of Periodic Limb Movements in Sleep Using Carbidopa/levodopa and Propoxyphene." *Sleep.* 1993; 16:717-723.

Ambrosetto C, Lugaresi E, Coccagna G, Tassinari CA. "Clinical and Polygraphic Remarks in the Restless Legs Syndrome." *Rivista Di Patologia Nervosa E Mentale.* 1965; 86:244-251.

American Sleep Disorders Association. "Periodic Limb Movement Disorder and Restless Legs Syndrome." In: *The International Classification of Sleep Disorders Diagnostic and Coding Manual.* Lawrence, Kansas: Allen Press, Inc. 1990; 65-71.

Ancoli-Israel S, Kripke DF, Mason W, Messin S. "Sleep Apnea and Nocturnal Myoclonus in a Senior Population." *Sleep.* 1981; 4:349-58.

Ancoli-Israel S, Kripke DF, Mason W, Kaplan OJ. "Sleep Apnea and Periodic Movements in an Aging Sample." *Journal of Gerontology.* 1985; 40:419-25.

Ancoli-Israel S, Seifert AR, Lemon M. "Thermal Biofeedback and Periodic Movements in Sleep: Patients' Subjective Reports and a Case Study." *Biofeedback Self Regulation.* 1986; 11:177-88.

Ancoli-Israel S, Kripke DF, Klauber MR, Mason WJ, Fell R, Kaplan O. "Periodic Limb Movements in Sleep in Community-Dwelling Elderly." *Sleep.* 1991; 14:496-500.

Atlas Task Force of the American Sleep Disorders Association. "Recording and Scoring Leg Movements." *Sleep.* 1993; 16:748-59.

Ausserwinkler M, Schmidt P. "Erfolgreiche Behandlung Des 'Restless Legs' - Syndroms Bei Chronishcher Niereninsuffizienz Mit Clonidin." *Schweizerische Medizinische Wochenschrift.* 1989; 119:184-186.

Ayers, Samuel, Jr. MD, FAPC and Milhan, Richard, M. "Restless Legs Syndrome: Response to Vitamin E." *Journal of Applied Nutrition.* 1993; 25:8-15.

Bastani B, Westervelt FB. "Effectiveness of Clonidine in Alleviating the Symptoms of 'Restless Legs.'" [letter] *American Journal of Kidney Diseases.* 1987; 10:326.

Becker PM, Jamieson AO, Brown WD. "Dopaminergic Agents in Restless Legs Syndrome and Periodic Limb Movements of Sleep: Response and Complications of Extended Treatment in 49 Cases." *Sleep.* 1993; 16:713-6.

Bixler EO, Kales A, Vela-Bueno A, Jacoby JA, Scarone S, Soldatos CR. "Nocturnal Myoclonus and Nocturnal Myoclonic Activity in a Normal Population." *Research Communications in Chemical Pathology and Pharmacology.* 1982; 36:129-40.

Bliwise DL, Petta D, Seidel W, Dement W. "Periodic Leg Movements During Sleep in the Elderly." *Archives of Gerontology and Geriatrics.* 1985; 4:273-81.

Bliwise DL, Carskadon MA, Dement WC. "Nightly Variation of Periodic Leg Movements in Sleep in Middle Aged and Elderly Individuals." *Archives of Gerontology and Geriatrics.* 1988; 7:273-9.

Bliwise DL, Ingham RH, Date ES, Dement WC. "Nerve Conduction and Creatinine Clearance in Aged People with Periodic Movements in Sleep." *Journal of Gerontology.* 1989; 44:164-7.

Boghen D, Peyronnard JM. "Myoclonus in Familial Restless Legs Syndrome." *Archives of Neurology.* 1976; 33:368-70.

Boghen D. "Successful Treatment of Restless Legs with Clonazepam." *Annals of Neurology.* 1980; 8:341.

Boghen D, Lamothe L, Elie R, Godbout R, Montplaisir J. "The Treatment of the Restless Legs Syndrome with Clonazepam: A Prospective Controlled Study." *Canadian Journal of Neurological Science.* 1986; 13:245-247.

Boivin DB, Montplaisir J, Poirier G. "The Effects of L-DOPA on Periodic Leg Movements and Sleep Organization in Narcolepsy." *Clinical Neuropharmacology.* 1989; 12:339-45.

Boivin DB, Montplaisir J, Lambert C. "Effects of Bromocriptine in Human Narcolepsy." *Clinical Neuropharmacology.* 1993a; 16:120-6.

Boivin DB, Lorrain D, Montplaisir J. "Effects of Bromocriptine on Periodic Limb Movements in Human Narcolepsy." *Neurology.* 1993b; 43: 2134-6.

Bonnet MH, Arand DL. "The Use of Triazolam in Older Patients with Periodic Leg Movements, Fragmented Sleep, and Daytime Sleepiness." *Journal of Gerontology.* 1990; 45:M139-44.

Bonnet MH, Arand DL. "Chronic Use of Triazolam in Patients with Periodic Leg Movements, Fragmented Sleep and Daytime Sleepiness." *Aging.* 1991; 3:313-24.

Bornstein B. "Restless Legs." *Psychiatric Neurology.* 1961; 141:165-201.

Botez, M.I., MD. "Folate Quiets Restless Legs.": *Understanding Vitamins and Minerals.* Rodale Press. 1994; 52.

Brenning R. "Growing Pains." *Acta Societatis Medicorum Upsaliensis.* 1960; 65:185-201.

Brodeur C, Montplaisir J, Godbout R, Marinier R. "Treatment of Restless Legs Syndrome and Periodic Movements During Sleep with L-DOPA: a Double-Blind, Controlled Study." *Neurology.* 1994; 38:1845-8.

Cadilhac J. "The EEG in Renal Insufficiency." In: Redmond A, editor. *Handbook of Electroencephalography and Clinical Neurophysiology.* Amsterdam: Elsevier, 1976: 15c51-15c69.

Callaghan N. "Restless Legs in Uraemic Neuropathy." *Neurology.* 1966; 16:359-361.

Cavatorta F, Vagge R, Solari P, Queirolo C. "Risultati Preliminari Con Clonidina Nella Sindrome Delle Gambe Senza Riposo in Due Pazienti Uremici Emodializzati." *Minerva Urologica & Nefrologica.* 1987; 39:93.

Coccagna G, Lugaresi E, Tassinari CA, Ambrosetto C. "La Sindrome Delle Gambe Senza Riposo (Restless Legs)." *Omnia Medica et Therapeutica.* 1966; 44:619-84.

Coccagna G, Lugaresi E. "Insomnia in the Restless Legs Syndrome." In: Gastaut H, Lugaresi E, Berti-Ceroni G, Coccagna G. (eds). *The Abnormalities of Sleep in Man.* Bologna: Aulo Gaggi Editore, 1968: 139-144.

Coccagna G, Montovani M, Brignani F, Manzini A. "Arterial Pressure Changes During Spontaneous Sleep in Man." *Electroencephalography and Clinical Neurophysiology.* 1971; 31:277-81.

Coccagna G, Lugaresi E. "Anxietas Tibiarum Und Nächtliche Myokloni." *EEG EMG Zeitschrift.* 1978; 9:155-160.

Coccagna G, Lugaresi E. "Restless Legs Syndrome and Nocturnal Myoclonus." *International Journal of Neurology.* 1981; 15:77-87.

Coccagna G. "Restless Legs Syndrome-Periodic Leg Movements in Sleep." In: Thorpy MJ, editor. *Handbook of Sleep Disorders.* New York: Marcel-Dekker Publishers, 1990:457-78.

Coleman RM, Pollak CP, Weitzman ED. "Periodic Movements in Sleep (Nocturnal Myoclonus): Relation to Sleep Disorders." *Annals of Neurology.* 1980; 8:416-21.

Coleman RM. "Periodic Movements in Sleep (Nocturnal Myoclonus) and Restless Legs Syndrome." In: Guilleminault C, editor. *Sleeping and Waking Disorders: Indications and Techniques.* Menlo Park, California: Addison-Wesley Publications, 1982a: 265-95.

Coleman RM, Bliwise DL, Sajben N, Boomkamp JGM, de Bruyn LM, Dement WC. "Daytime Sleepiness in Patients with Periodic Movements in Sleep." *Sleep.* 1982b; 5 (suppl):S191-202.

Coleman RM, Bliwise DL, Sajben N, de Bruyn L, Boomkamp A, Menn ME, Dement WC. "Epidemiology of Periodic Movements During Sleep." In: Guilleminault C, Lugaresi E, editors. *Sleep/wake Disorders; Natural History, Epidemiology, and Long-Term Evolution.* New York: Raven Press, 1983; 217-29.

Culpepper W, Badia P, Shaffer J. "Time-of-Night Patterns in PLMS Activity." *Sleep.* 1992; 15:306-311.

Dickel MJ, Mosko SS. "Morbidity Cut-Offs for Sleep Apnea and Periodic Leg Movements in Predicting Subjective Complaints in Seniors." *Sleep.* 1990; 13:155-166.

de Groen JHM, Kamphuisen HAC. "Periodic Nocturnal Myoclonus in a Patient with Hyperekplexia (Startle Disease)." *Journal of Neurology Science.* 1978; 38:207-13.

Doghramji K, Browman CP, Gaddy JR, Walsh JK. "Triazolam Diminishes Daytime Sleepiness and Sleep Fragmentation in Patients with Periodic Leg Movements in Sleep." *Journal of Clinical Psychopharmacology.* 1991; 11:284-90.

Dzvonik ML, Kripke DF, Klauber M, Ancoli-Israel S. "Body Position Changes and Periodic Movements in Sleep." *Sleep.* 1986; 9:484-91.

Ehrenberg BL. "Valproate for Periodic Limb Movements of Sleep." *EEG Clinical Neurophysiology.* 1991; 79:65P.

Ehrenberg B, Eisensehr I, Walters A. "Influence of Valproate on Sleep and Periodic Limb Movements Disorder." *Sleep Research.* 1995; 24: 227.

Ekbom KA. "Asthenia Crurum Paraesthetica (Irritable Legs)." *Acta Medica Scandinavica.* 1944; 118:197-209.

Ekbom KA. "Restless Legs: A Clinical Study." *Acta Medica Scandinavica.* 1945; 158(Suppl.):1-123.

Ekbom KA. "Restless Legs." *Journal of the American Medical Association.* 1946; 131:481.

Ekbom KA. "Restless Legs – A Report of 70 New Cases." *Acta Medica Scandinavica.* 1950; 246(Suppl.):64-68.

Ekbom KA. "Restless Legs Syndrome." *Neurology.* 1960; 10:868-873.

Ekbom KA. "Restless Legs in Amputees." *Acta Medica Scandinavica.* 1961; 169:419-421.

Ekbom K. "Restless Legs Syndrome after Partial Gastrectomy." *Acta Neurologica Scandinavica.* 1966; 42:79-89.

Ekbom K. "Restless Legs." In: Vinken PJ, Bruyn GW, editors. *Handbook of Clinical Neurology.* Amsterdam: North Holland Publishing Company, 1970; 311-20.

Eqawa I, Sugita Y, Teshima Y, et al. "A Polysomnographic Study of Restless Legs Syndrome in Patients Undergoing Hemodialysis Treatment." *Sleep Research.* 1987; 16:330.

Fry JM, Di Phillipo MA, Pressman MR. "Periodic Leg Movements in Sleep Following Treatment of Obstructive Sleep Apnea with Nasal Continuous Positive Airway Pressure." *Chest.* 1989; 96:89-91.

Godbout R, Montplaisir J, Poirier G. "Epidemiological Data in Familial Restless Legs Syndrome." *Sleep Research.* 1987; 16:338.

Godbout R, Montplaisir J, Bédard MA, Boivin D, Lapierre O. "Fundamental and Clinical Neuropharmacology of Sleep Disorders: Restless Legs Syndrome with Periodic Movements in Sleep and Narcolepsy." In: Montplaisir J, Godbout R, editors. *Sleep and Biological Rhythms: Basic Mechanisms and Application to Psychiatry.* New York: Oxford University Press, 1990; 219-36.

Gorman C, Dyck P, Pearson J. "Symptoms of Restless Legs." *Archives of Internal Medicine.* 1965; 115:155-160.

Guilleminault C, Flagg W. "Effects of Baclofen on Sleep-Related Periodic Leg Movements." *Annals of Neurology.* 1984; 15:234-239.

Guilleminault C, Cetel M, Philip P. "Dopaminergic Treatment of Restless Legs and Rebound Phenomenon." *Neurology.* 1993; 43:445.

Handwerker JV, Palmer RF. "Clonidine in the Treatment of 'Restless Legs' Syndrome." *New England Journal of Medicine.* 1985; 313:1228-1229.

Hartman P, Scrima L. "Muscle Activity in the Legs (MAL) Associated with Frequent Arousals in Narcoleptics and OSA Patients." *Clinical EEG.* 1986; 17:181-186.

Hening W, Walters A, Kavey N, Gidro-Frank S, FS. Cote L. "Dyskinesias While Awake and Periodic Movements of Sleep in Restless Legs Syndrome: Treatment with Opioids." *Neurology.* 1986; 36:1363-1366.

Hening WA, Chokroverty S, Walters AS. "Presence of a Biphasic Cortical Prepotential Before Leg Jerks in the Restless Legs Syndrome." *Sleep Research.* 1990; 19:235.

Hening W, Chokroverty S, Rolleri M, Walters A. "The Cortical Premovement Potentials of Restless Legs Syndrome Jerks: Differences in Potentials Before Simulated Versus Symptomatic Jerks." *Sleep Research.* 1991; 20:255.

Hickey K, Walters A, Hening W. "Hyperactivity and 'Growing Pains' as Possible Misdiagnoses in Young-Age Onset Restless Legs Syndrome." *Sleep Research.* 1992; 21:209.

Hirshkowitz M, Karacan I, Arcasoy MO, Acik G, Williams RL. "The Prevalence of Periodic Limb Movements During Sleep in Men with Erectile Dysfunction." *Biological Psychiatry.* 1989; 26:541-4.

Holley JL, Nespor S, Rault R. "Characterizing Sleep Disorders in Chronic Hemodialysis Patients." *ASAIO Transactions.* 1991; 37:M456-7.

Holley JL, Nespor S, Rault R. "A Comparison of Reported Sleep Disorders in Patients on Chronic Hemodialysis and Continuous Peritoneal Dialysis." *American Journal of Kidney Diseases.* 1992; 19:156-161.

Horiguchi J, Inami Y, Sasaki A, Nishimatsu O, Sugekawa T. "Periodic Leg Movements in Sleep with Restless Legs Syndrome: Effect of Clonazepam Treatment." *Japanese Journal of Psychiatry and Neurology.* 1992; 46:727-32.

Iannaccone S, Zucconi M, Marchettini P, Ferini-Strambi L, Nemni R, Quattrini A, Palazzi S, Lacerenza M, Formaglio F, Smirne S. "Evidence of Peripheral Axonal Neuropathy in Primary Restless Legs Syndrome." *Movement Disorders.* 1995; 10:2-9.

Johnson W, Walters A, Lehner T, Coccagna G, Ehrenberg B, Lazzarini A, et al. "Affecteds Only Linkage Analysis of Autosomal Dominant Restless Legs Syndrome." *Sleep Research.* 1992; 21:214.

Kanter, A. "The Effect of Sclerotherapy on Restless Legs Syndrome." *Journal of Dermatological Surgery.* 1995; 21:328-32.

Kavey N, Walters A, Hening W, Gidro-Frank S. "Opioid Treatment of Periodic Movements in Sleep in Patients Without Restless Legs." *Neuropeptides.* 1988; 11:181-184.

Kotagal S, Rathnow SR, Chu JY, O'Connor DM, Cross J, Sterneck RL. "Nocturnal Myoclonus – A Sleep Disturbance in Children with Leukemia." *Developmental Medicine and Child Neurology.* 1985; 27:124-7.

Kovacevic-Ristanovic R, Cartwright RD, Lloyd S. "Nonpharmacologic Treatment of Periodic Leg Movements in Sleep." *Archives of Physical Medicine & Rehabilitation.* 1991; 72:385-9.

Kripke DF, Ancoli-Israel S, Okudaira N. "Sleep Apnea and Nocturnal Myoclonus in the Elderly." *Neurobiology of Aging.* 1982; 3:329-36.

LaBan MM, Viola SL, Femminineo AF, Taylor RS. "Restless Legs Syndrome Associated with Diminished Cardiopulmonary Compliance and Lumbar Spinal Stenosis-A Motor Concomitant of 'Vesper's Curse.'" *Archives of Physical Medicine & Rehabilitation.* 1990; 71:384-388.

Lang, A. "Patient Perception of Tics and Other Movement Disorders." *Neurology.* 1991; 41:223-228.

Lang AE. "Akathisia and the Restless Legs Syndrome." In: Jankovic J, Tolosa E (eds). *Parkinson's Disease and Movement Disorders, Chapter 23.* Baltimore, MD: Williams & Wilkins, Second Edition 1993: 399-418.

Lavigne G, Montplaisir J. "Restless Legs Syndrome and Sleep Bruxism: Prevalence and Association among Canadians." *Sleep.* 1994; 17: 739-743.

Lipinski, Jr. JF, Hudson JI, Cunningham SL, Aizley HG, Keck PE, Mallya G, Aranow RB, Lukas SE. "Polysomnographic Characteristics of Neuroleptic-Induced Akathisia." *Clinical Neuropharmacology.* 1991; 14:413-9.

Lorrain D, Montplaisir J. "The Forced Immobilization Test: An Objective Method of Quantifying Severity of the Restless Legs Syndrome." *Sleep Research.* 1990; 19:247.

Lugaresi E, Tassinari CA, Coccagna G, Ambrosetto C. "Particularites Cliniques et Polygraphiques du Syndrome D'impatience Des Membres Inferieurs." *Rivista Di Neurologia.* 1965a; 113:545-55.

Lugaresi E, Coccagna G, Tassinari CA, Ambrosetto C. "Relievi Poligrafici Sui Fenomeni Motori Nella Sindrome Delle Gambe Senza Riposo." *Rivista Di Neurologia.* 1965b; 35:550-61.

Lugaresi E, Coccagna G, Gambi D, Berti-Ceroni G, Poppi M. "A Propos De Quelques Manifestations Nocturnes Myocloniques (Nocturnal Myoclonus De Symonds)." *Revue Neurologique.* 1966; 115:547-55.

Lugaresi E, Berti-Ceroni G, Coccagna G, Ambrosetto C. "Mioclonie Notturne Sintomatiche." *Systema Nervoso.* 1967; 19:71-80.

Lugaresi E, Coccagna G, Berti-Ceroni G, Ambrosetto C. "Restless Legs Syndrome and Nocturnal Myoclonus." In: Gastaut H, Lugaresi E, Berti-Ceroni G, Coccagna G, editors. *The Abnormalities of Sleep in Man.* Bologna: Aulo Gaggi Editore, 1968; 285-94.

Lugaresi E, Coccagna G, Montovani M, Lebrun R. "Some Periodic Phenomena Arising During Drowsiness and Sleep in Man." *Electroencephalogr Clin Neurophysiol.* 1972; 32:701-5.

Lugaresi E, Cirignotta F, Coccagna G, Montagna P. "Nocturnal Myoclonus and Restless Legs Syndrome." In: Fahn S, Marsden CD, Van Woert M, editors. *Advances in Neurology: Myoclonus.* New York: Raven Press, 1986; 43:295-307.

Lundvall O, Abom PE, Holm R. "Carbamazepine in Restless Legs: A Controlled Pilot Study." *European Journal of Clinical Pharmacology.* 1983; 25:323-4.

Lutz EG. "Restless Legs, Anxiety and Caffeinism." *Journal of Clinical Psychiatry.* 1978; 39:693-698.

Marsden CD, Hallet M, Fahn S. "The Nosology and Pathophysiology of Myoclonas." In: Marsden CD, Fahn S, eds. *Movement Disorders.* London: Butterworths, 1982; 196-248.

Martinelli P, Pazzaglia P, Montagna P, Coccagna G, Rizzuto N, Simonati S, Lugaresi E. "Stiffman Associated with Nocturnal Myoclonus and Epilepsy." *Journal of Neurology, Neurosurgery, and Psychiatry.* 1978; 41:458-62.

Martinelli P, Coccagna G, Lugaresi E. "Nocturnal Myoclonus, Restless Legs Syndrome, and Abnormal Electrophysiological Findings." *Annals of Neurology.* 1987; 2:515.

Matthews WB. "Treatment of the Restless Legs Syndrome with Clonazepam." *British Medical Journal.* 1979; 281:751.

McParland P, Pearce JM. "Restless Legs Syndrome in Pregnancy. Case Reports." *Clinical and Experimental Obstetrics & Gynecology.* 1990; 17:5-6.

Moldofsky H, Tullis C, Lue FA, Quance G, Davidson J. "Sleep Related Myoclonus in Rheumatic Pain Modulation Disorder and in Excessive Daytime Somnolence." *Psychosomatic Medicine.* 1984; 46:145-51.

Moldolfsky H, Tullis C, Quance G, Lue FA. "Nitrazepam for Periodic Movements in Sleep (Sleep Related Myoclonus)." *Canadian Journal of Neurological Science.* 1986a; 13:52-54.

Moldofsky H, Tullis C, Lue FA. "Sleep Related Myoclonus in Rheumatic Pain Modulation Disorder (Fibrositis Syndrome)." *Journal of Rheumatology.* 1986b; 13:614-7.

Montagna P, Coccagna G, Cirignotta F, Lugaresi E. "Familial Restless Legs Syndrome: Long-Term Follow-up." In: Guilleminault C, Lugaresi E, editors. *Sleep/Wake Disorders: Natural History, Epidemiology, and Long-Term Evolution.* New York, NY: Raven Press. 1983; 231-5.

Montagna P, Sassoli de Bianchi L, Zucconi M, Cirignotta F, Lugaresi E. "Clonazepam and Vibration in Restless Legs Syndrome." *Acta Neurologica Scandinavica.* 1984; 69:428-430.

Montplaisir J, Godbout R, Boghen D, De Champlain J, Young SN, Lapierre G, Ing M. "Familial Restless Legs with Periodic Movements in Sleep: Electrophysiologic, Biochemical and Pharmacologic Study." *Neurology.* 1985; 35:130-4.

Montplaisir J, Godbout R, Poirier G, Bedard MA. "Restless Legs Syndrome and Periodic Movements in Sleep: Physiopathology and Treatment with L-DOPA." *Clinical Neuropharmacology.* 1986; 9: 456-468.

Montplaisir J, Lorrain D, Godbout R. "Restless Legs Syndrome and Periodic Leg Movements in Sleep: the Primary Role of Dopaminergic Mechanism." *European Neurology.* 1991; 31:41-3.

Montplaisir J, Lapierre O, Warnes H, Pelletier G. "The Treatment of the Restless Legs Syndrome With or Without Periodic Leg Movements in Sleep." *Sleep.* 1992; 15:391-5.

Montplaisir J, Lapierre O, Lavigne G. "The Restless Legs Syndrome: A Condition Associated with Periodic or Aperiodic Slowing of the EEG." *Neurophysiologie Clinique.* 1994a; 24:131-40.

Montplaisir J, Godbout R, Pelletier G, Warnes H. "Restless Legs Syndrome and Periodic Limb Movements During Sleep." In: Kryger MH, Roth T, Dement WC, editors. *Principles and Practice of Sleep Medicine.* Philadelphia: WB Saunders, 1994b; 589-597.

Montplaisir J, Boucher S, Gosselin A, Gaétan P, LaVigne G. "The Restless Legs Syndrome: Evening vs. Morning Restlessness." *Sleep Research.* 1995; 24:302.

Montplaisir J, Boucher S, Poirier G, Lavigne G, Lapierre O, Lesperance P. "Clinical Polysomnographic and Genetic Characteristics of Restless Legs Syndrome: A Study of 133 Patients Diagnosed with New Standard Criteria." *Movement Disorders.* 1996; submitted.

Morgan LK. Restless limbs: "A Commonly Overlooked Symptom Controlled by Valium." *The Medical Journal of Australia.* 1967; 2:589-594.

Mosko SS, Nudleman KL. "Somatosensory and Brainstem Auditory Evoked Responses in Sleep-Related Periodic Leg Movements." *Sleep.* 1986; 9:399-404.

Mosko SS, Dickel MJ, Ashurst J. "Night to Night Variability in Sleep Apnea and Sleep Related Periodic Leg Movements in the Elderly." *Sleep.* 1988a; 11:340-8.

Mosko SS, Dickel MJ, Paul T, La Tour T, Dhillon S, Ghanim A, Sassin JF. "Sleep Apnea and Sleep-Related Periodic Leg Movements in Community Resident Seniors." *Journal of the American Geriatrics Society.* 1988b; 36:502-8.

Nishimatsu OI, Horiguchi J, Inami Y, Innami T, Sasaki A, Kondo K. "Nocturnal Myoclonus in a Patient with Neuroleptic-Induced Akathisia." *Japanese Journal of Psychiatry and Neurology.* 1992; 46:121-6.

Oshtory MA, Vijayan N. "Clonazepam Treatment of Insomnia Due to Sleep Myoclonus." *Archives of Neurology.* 1980; 37:119-120.

Passouant P, Cadilhac J, Baldy-Moulinier M, Mion CH. "Etude du Sommeil Nocturne Chez Des Uremiques Chroniques Soumis a Une Epuration Extrarenale." *Electroencephalography and Clinical Neurophysiology.* 1970; 29:441-9.

Peled R, Lavie P. "Double-Blind Evaluation of Clonazepam on Periodic Leg Movements in Sleep." *Journal of Neurology, Neurosurgery, and Psychiatry.* 1987; 50:1679-81.

Pelletier G, Lorrain D, Montplaisir J. "Sensory and Motor Components of the Restless Legs Syndrome." *Neurology.* 1992; 42:1663-6.

Picchietti DL, Walters AS. "Attention Deficit Hyperactivity Disorder and Periodic Limb Movement Disorder in Childhood." *Sleep Research.* 1994; 23:303.

Picchietti DL, Walters AS. "Restless Legs Syndrome: Parent-Child Pairs." *Sleep Research.* 1995; 24: 319.

Pollmächer T, Schulz H. "Periodic Leg Movements (PLM) — Their Relationship to Sleep Stages." *Sleep.* 1993; 16:572-7.

Popoviciu L, Asgian B, DeLast Popoviciu "Detal-Clinical EEG, Electomyographic and Polysonnographic Studies in Restless Legs Syndrome Caused by Magnesium Deficiency." *Romanian Journal of Neurology and Psychiatry.* 1993; 31: 55-61

Read DJ, Feest TG, Nassim MA. "Clonazepam: Effective Treatment for Restless Legs Syndrome in Uraemia." *British Medical Journal.* 1981; 283:885-886.

Roehrs T, Zorick F, Sicklesteel J, Wittig R, Roth T. "Age-Related Sleep-Wake Disorders at a Sleep Disorders Center." *Journal of the American Geriatrics Society.* 1983; 31:364-70.

Roger SD, Harris DCH, Stewart JH. "Possible Relation Between Restless Legs and Anemia in Renal Dialysis Patients." *Lancet* 1991; I:1551.

Rosen et al. "Physician Education in Sleep and Sleep Disorders: A National Survey of U.S. Medical Schools." *Sleep. 1994;* 16(3):249-254.

Salvi F, Montagna P, Plasmati R, Rubboli G, Cirignotta F, Veilleux M, Lugaresi E, Tassinari CA. "Restless Legs Syndrome and Nocturnal Myoclonus: Initial Clinical Manifestation of Familial Amyloid Polyneuropathy." *Journal of Neurology, Neurosurgery, and Psychiatry.* 1990; 53:522-5.

Sandyk R, Bernick G, Lee SM, Stern LZ, Iacono RP, Bamford CR. "L-DOPA in Uremic Patients with Restless Legs Syndrome." *International Journal of Neuroscience.* 1987a; 35:233-235.

Sandyk R, Bamford CR, Gillman MA. "Opiates in the Restless Legs Syndrome." *International Journal of Neuroscience.* 1987b; 36:99-104.

Schmidt HS, Wise HA. "Significance of Impaired Penile Tumescence and Associated Polysomnographic Abnormalities in the Impotent Patient." *Journal of Urology.* 1981; 126:348-52.

Scrima L. "An Etiology of Narcolepsy-Cataplexy and a Proposed Cataplexy Neuromechanism." *International Journal of Neuroscience.* 1981; 15:69-86.

Scrima L, "Gamma-Hydroxybutyrate (GHB) Treated Narcolepsy Patients Continue to Report Cataplexy Controlled For Up to Five Years." *Sleep Research.* 1992; 21:262.

Scrima L, Hartman P, Johnson FH, Hiller FC. "Efficacy of Gamma-Hydroxybutyrate (GHB) vs. Placebo in Treating Narcolepsy-Cataplexy: Double Blind Measures." *Biological Psychiatry.* 1989; 26:331-343.

Scrima L. "Isolated REM Sleep Facilitates Recall of Complex Associative Information." *Psychophysiology.* 1982; 19:252-259.

Scrima L, Hartman P, Johnson FH, Thomas EE, Hiller FC. "The Effects of Gama-Hydroxybutyrate on the Sleep of Narcolepsy Patients: A Double Blind Study." *Sleep.* 1990; 13(6):479-490.

Scrima L, Stedman D, Thomas G, Johnson F, Hiller FC. "Arousals After Alcolhol Ingestion in Asyptomatic Nocturnal Myoclonus Subjects." *Sleep Research.* 1986; 15:168.

Shafor R. "Prevalence of Abnormal Lumbo-Sacral Spine Imaging in Patients with Insomnia Associated Restless Legs, Periodic Leg Movements in Sleep." *Sleep Research.* 1991; 20:396.

Smith RC. "Relationship of Periodic Movements in Sleep (Nocturnal Myoclonus) and the Babinski Sign." *Sleep.* 1985; 8:239-43.

Smith RC. "Comparison of Babinski-Like Response in Periodic Movements in Sleep (Nocturnal Myoclonus)." *Biological Psychiatry.* 1987; 22:1271-3.

Smith RC, Gouin PR, Minkley P, Lyles J, Van Egeren L, Adams T, Shaffer D, Hulce V. "Periodic Limb Movement Disorder Is Associated with Normal Motor Conduction Latencies When Studied by Central Magnetic Stimulation–Successful Use of a New Technique." *Sleep.* 1992; 15:312-8.

Staedt J, Stoppe G, Kogler A, Munz D, Riemann H, Emrich D, Ruther E. "Dopamine D2 Receptor Alteration in Patients with Periodic Movements in Sleep (Nocturnal Myoclonus)." *Journal of Neural Transmission.* 1993; 93:71-4.

Stark RJ. "Reversible Myoclonus with Uraemia." *British Medical Journal.* 1981; 282:1119-20.

Steiner JC. "Clonidine Helps in Restless Legs Syndrome." *Neurology.* 1987; 37 (Suppl.):278.

Stoller, Melissa Kaleta, M.A., Department of Anthropology, The University of Chicago, Chicago, Illinois. Reprinted from *Clinical Therapeutics,* 1994; Vol. 16, No. 5, Excerpt Medica, Inc.

Symonds CP. "Nocturnal Myoclonus." *Journal of Neurology, Neurosurgery, and Psychiatry.* 1953; 16:166-71.

Telstad W, Sorensen O, Larsen S, Lillevold PE, Stensrud P, Nyberg-Hansen R. "Treatment of the Restless Legs Syndrome with Carbamazepine: A Double-Blind Study." *British Medical Journal.* 1984; 288:444-446.

Trenkwalder C, Bucher SF, Oertel WH, Proeckl D, Plendl H, Paulus W. "Bereitschaftspotential in Idiopathic and Symptomatic Restless Legs Syndrome." *Electroencephalography and Clinical Neurophysiology.* 1993; 89:95-103.

Trenkwalder C, Stiasny K, Pollmacher Th, Wetter Th, Schwarz J, Kohnen R, Kazenwadel J, Kruger HP, Ramm S, Kunzel M, Oertel WH. "L-DOPA Therapy of Uremic and Idiopathic Restless Legs Syndrome: A Double-Blind Crossover Trial." *Sleep.* 1995a; 18: 681-688.

Trenkwalder C, Walters AS, Hening W, Campbell S, Rahman K, Chokroverty S. "Circadian Rhythm of Patients with the Idiopathic Restless Legs Syndrome." *Sleep Research.* 1995b; 24:360.

Trzepacz PT, Violette EJ, Sateia MJ. "Response to Opioids in Three Patients with Restless Legs Syndrome." *American Journal of Psychiatry.* 1984; 141:993-995.

Uchihara T, Ichikawa T, Furukawa T, Tsukagoshi H. "Myoclonus with Burning Sensation in Legs That Remits with Sympathetic Blockade." *Journal of the Neurological Sciences.* 1990; 100:161-4.

von Scheele C. "Levodopa in Restless Legs." *Lancet.* 1986; 2:426-427.

von Scheele C, Kempi V. "Long-Term Effect of Dopaminergic Drugs in Restless Legs." *Archives of Neurology.* 1990; 47:1223-1224.

Wagner ML, Walters AS, Coleman RG, Hening WA, Grasing K, Chokroverty S. "A Randomized Double-Blind Placebo Controlled Study of Clonidine in Restless Legs Syndrome." *Sleep.* 1996; 19:52-58.

Walters A, Hening W, Chokroverty S, Fahn S. "Opioid Responsiveness in Patients with Neuroleptic-Induced Akathisia." *Movement Disorders.* 1986a; I: 119-127.

Walters A, Hening W, Cote L, Fahn S. "Dominantly Inherited Restless Legs with Myoclonus and Periodic Movements of Sleep: A Syndrome Related to the Endogenous Opiates?" *Advances in Neurology.* 1986b; 43:309-19.

Walters AS, Hening W. "Clinical Presentation and Neuropharmacology of Restless Legs Syndrome." *Clinical Neuropharmacology.* 1987; 10:225-37. Erratum in 1987; 10:482.

Walters AS, Hening W, Chokroverty S. "Frequent Occurrence of Myoclonus While Awake and at Rest, Body Rocking and Marching-in-Place in a Subpopulation of Patients with Restless Legs Syndrome." *Acta Neurologica Scandinavica.* 1988a; 77:418-21.

Walters AS, Hening WA, Kavey N, Chokroverty S, Gidro-Frank S. "A Double-Blind Crossover Trial of Bromocriptine and Placebo in Restless Legs Syndrome." *Annals of Neurology.* 1988b; 24:455-8.

Walters AS, Hening W. "Opioids a Better Treatment for Acute than Tardive Akathisia: Possible Role for the Endogenous Opiate System in Neuroleptic-Induced Akathisia." *Medical Hypotheses.* 1989; 28:1-2.

Walters AS, Picchietti D, Hening W, Lazzarini A. "Variable Expressivity in Familial Restless Legs Syndrome." *Archives of Neurology.* 1990; 47:1219-20.

Walters AS, Hening WA, Chokroverty S. "Review and Videotape Recognition of Idiopathic Restless Legs Syndrome." *Movement Disorders.* 1991a; 6:105-10.

Walters AS, Hening W, Rubinstein M, Chokroverty S. "A Clinical and Polysomnographic Comparison of Neuroleptic-Induced Akathisia and the Idiopathic Restless Legs Syndrome." *Sleep.* 1991b; 14:339-45.

Walters A, Johnson W, Lehner T, Coccagna G, Ehrenberg B, Lazzarini A, et al. "Linkage Analysis of Autosomal Dominant Restless Legs Syndrome." *Movement Disorders.* 1992; 7:301-302.

Walters AS, Wagner ML, Hening WA, Grasing K, Mills R, Chokroverty S, Kavey N. "Successful Treatment of the Idiopathic Restless Legs Syndrome in a Randomized Double-Blind Trial of Oxycodone Versus Placebo." *Sleep.* 1993; 16:327-32.

Walters AS, Picchietti D, Ehrenberg B, Wagner M. "Restless Legs Syndrome in Childhood and Adolescence." *Pediatric Neurology.* 1994; 11: 241-245.

Walters AS. "Group Organizer and Correspondent-International Restless Legs Syndrome Study Group. Toward a Better Definition of the Idiopathic Restless Legs Syndrome." *Movement Disorders.* 1995a; 10: 634-642.

Walters AS. "Periodic Limb Movements." In: Aldrich MS, ed. *Neurobase (a computer based program in Neurology): Sleep Disorders Section.* La Jolla, CA: Arbor Publishing, 1995b.

Walters AS, Trenkwalder C, Hening WA, Chokroverty S, Dhawan V, Eidelberg D. "Fluorodeoxyglucose PET Scanning in 5 Patients with Restless Legs Syndrome." *Sleep Research.* 1995c; 24: 360.

Walters AS, Trenkwalder C, Hening W, Chokroverty S, Rahman K. "Circadian Rhythm of the Restless Legs Syndrome." *Neurology.* 1995d; 45 (Suppl 4.): A 285.

Walters AS, Hickey K, Maltzman J, Verrico T, Joseph D, Hening W, Wilson V, Chokroverty S. "A Questionnaire Study of 138 Patients with Restless Legs Syndrome: The 'Nightwalkers' Survey." *Neurology.* 1996; 46:92-95.

Ware JC, Pittard JT, Blumoff RL. "Treatment of Sleep Related Myoclonus with an Alpha-Receptor Blocker." *Sleep Research.* 1981; 10:242.

Ware JC, Brown FW, Moorad PJ, Pittard JT, Murphy M, Franklin D. "Nocturnal Myoclonus and Tricyclic Antidepressants." *Sleep Research.* 1984; 13:72.

Ware JC. "Nocturnal Myoclonus: Possible Mediation by the Sympathetic Nervous System." *Sleep Research.* 1985; 14:247.

Ware JC, Blumoff R, Pittard JT. "Peripheral Vasoconstriction in Patients with Sleep Related Periodic Leg Movements." *Sleep.* 1988; 11:182-7.

Watanabe S, Sakai K, Ono Y, Seino H, Naito H. "Alternating Periodic Leg Movement Induced by Spinal Anesthesia in an Elderly Male." *Anesthesia and Analgesia.* 1987; 66:1031-2.

Watanabe S, Ono A, Naito H. "Periodic Leg Movements During Either Epidural or Spinal Anesthesia in an Elderly Man Without Sleep-Related (Nocturnal) Myoclonus." *Sleep.* 1990; 13:262-6.

Wechsler LR, Stakes JW, Shahani BT, Busis NA. "Periodic Leg Movements of Sleep (Nocturnal Myoclonus): An Electrophysiological Study." *Annals of Neurology.* 1986; 19:168-73.

Wersäll J. "Restless Legs." *Svenska Läk-Tidn.* 1952; 49:2032-2034.

Willis T. *The London Practice of Physick.* 1st ed. London: Thomas Basset and William Crooke, 1685; 404.

Yamakawa T, Yokota T, Suga M. "A Case of Chronic Inflammatory Demyelinating Polyradiculoneuropathy with Nocturnal Myoclonus." *Clinical Neurology.* 1990; 30:1017-19.

Yamashiro Y, Kryger MH. "Acute Effect of Nasal Cpap on Periodic Limb Movements Associated with Breathing Disorders During Sleep." *Sleep.* 1994; 17:172-3

Yoakam, Robert. "Night Walkers. Do Your Legs Seem to Have a Life of Their Own?" *Modern Maturity.* 1994; Vol. 37, No. 5:54.

Yokota T, Hirose K, Tanabe H, Tsukagoshi H. "Sleep-Related Periodic Leg Movements (Nocturnal Myoclonus) Due to Spinal Cord Lesion." *Journal of the Neurological Sciences.* 1991; 104:13-18.

Zoe A, Wagner ML, Walters AS. "High Dose Clonidine in a Case of Restless Legs Syndrome." *The Annals of Pharmacotherapy.* 1994; 28: 878-881.

Zucconi M, Coccagna G, Petronelli R, Gerardi R, Mondini S, Cirignotta F. "Nocturnal Myoclonus in Restless Legs Syndrome: Effect of Carbamazepine Treatment." *Functional Neurology.* 1989; 4:263-71.

Appendix 4

Glossary

ABSM - American Board of Sleep Medicine
ADHD - Attention Deficit Hyperactivity Disorder
APSS - Associaton of Professional Sleep Societies
ASDA - American Sleep Disorders Association
EDS - excessive daytime sleepiness
EEG - electroencephalogram
FIT - forced immobilization test
GHB - gamma-hydroxybutyrate
mg - milligram
MS - Multiple Sclerosis
MSLT - multiple sleep latency test
NIA - neuroleptic induced akathisia
NIH - National Institutes of Health
NLM - National Library of Medicine
NM - nocturnal myoclonus
NORD - National Organization for Rare Diseases
PD - Parkinson's Disease
PET - Positron Emisssion Tomography
PLM - Periodic Limb Movements
PLMD - Periodic Limb Movement Disorder
PLMS - Periodic Limb Movements in Sleep
prn - as needed
REM - rapid eye movement
RLS - Restless Legs Syndrome
RLSF - Restless Legs Syndrome Foundation
SIT - suggested immobilization test
SRUP - serotonin re-uptake blockers

Appendix 5

Index